Vegetarian Cooking for Diabetics

Patricia Mozzer

Revised Edition

The Book Publishing Company • Summertown, Tennessee 38483

Author: Patricia Mozzer

Photography: Michael Bonnickson

Food Stylist: Louise Hagler

Editors: Dorothy Bates Nutritional Consultant:
    Louise Hagler Jamie Pope-Cordle, M.S., R.D.

Design: Louise Hagler
    Cynthia Holzapfel
    Richard Martin

Mozzer, Patricia
    Vegetarian cooking for diabetics.

    Includes index.
    1.Diabetes—Diet therapy—Recipes.   2.Cookery
(Vegetables)   I.Title.
RC662.M69   1988   641.5'6314   87-35235
ISBN 0-913990-59-0

On the cover, Sesame-Cornmeal Biscuits, p. 65, Tofu Salad I, p. 71, The Islander, p. 126, Millet with Peas & Sesame, p. 99, Tofu Lasagne, p. 96

In appreciation....
We all know that being a diabetic is difficult at best. A large part of the difficulty is adjusting to the eating regimen. Keeping track of fats, carbo-hydrates and proteins can be a real challenge. In my case, the change in eating habits had been for the better. I am much more aware of the nutritional value of that which I eat. About the time I was diagnosed a diabetic, I was undergoing the transition from meat eater to vegetarian. The more that Pat and I read about diabetic diets, the clearer it became that a vegetarian meal plan could be very beneficial. We soon learned that there were no diabetic vegetarian cookbooks available. There was plenty of raw data to support our theory, but no one had combined the two subjects. Pat decided to compile her recipes so that they might be shared with other diabetics. At the beginning this seemed like a simple project! The under-taking has grown until it became this complete manual for diabetic vegetarians. My part in the project has been fun. I try out all the recipes. They are all great. Now all diabetics can try vegetarian dishes without all the guesswork about calories. This book is a great step in devising diabetic meal plans. I hope that everyone enjoys these recipes as much as I do. Many thanks to Pat.

Ken Bastura

TABLE OF CONTENTS

Foreword

Diabetes mellitus affects about 11 million Americans and is a major cause for damage to the eyes, kidneys and blood vessels. Proper care of diabetes is essential because there is no known cure and good management reduces all the associated problems.

Proper diet is the cornerstone for any successful diabetes management plan. Generous intakes of starchy foods rich in fiber are essential for good diabetes control. Recommended foods include all types of grain products, cereals, vegetables, beans and lentils, and fruits. Almost everyone, with or without diabetes, would benefit from increasing the intake of these plant foods and decreasing the intake of high-fat meat and dairy products.

Recommendations for diet for diabetic individuals have changed radically in the past decade. Instead of restricting intake of sugars and starches, most experts strongly urge that diabetic individuals eat less fat (such as high-fat meats, dairy products, and bakery products made with lots of shortening, butter or oil).

Recently the American Diabetes Association recommended that most diabetic individuals should have a generous carbohydrate intake (50-60% of calories from starches and simple carbohydrates) and a liberal fiber intake (30-50 grams per day) while limiting the intake of fat to less than 30% of calories. The vegetarian meal plans outlined in this book follow these guidelines for healthy eating.

Incorporating more grains (wheat, barley, oats, etc.), more vegetables, more beans and lentils, and more fruits into the diet provides health advantages for almost everyone. These diet changes lower blood fats (including cholesterol), decrease blood pressure, assist in weight management, and decrease the risk for heart attacks and strokes.

Ms. Mozzer offers practical guidelines to help diabetic individuals incorporate more vegetarian items into their diet. Although I am not vegetarian, I follow a prudent diet that is vegetarian in orientation for breakfast and lunch each day and have fish, poultry or meat at dinner only three or four times weekly.

Although I do not have diabetes, I follow a prudent diet similar to the one I prescribe for the diabetic individuals in my practice. This creative book presents many innovative recipes my family will be enjoying. Your health may benefit from adapting some of the practices outlined in this book.

James W. Anderson, M.D.
Professor of Medicine and
Clinical Nutrition
University of Kentucky
Lexington, Kentucky

Introduction

This book is for diabetics and their families who are interested in either varying their diet to include vegetarian meals, or who want to make a complete change to vegetarianism. When my husband, Ken, was diagnosed as being diabetic, we had been following a vegetarian diet for about two years. We wanted to keep eating these foods, but could find little information on how to fit vegetarian combinations into a diabetic's exchange system diet. Ken had been given a diet which allowed him a certain number of calories and which defined how much and what food from each food group he should have per day. One of the groups was the "meat" group, which listed how much of what meats, eggs and cheese should be eaten at a meal. We knew that combinations of legumes, grains, nuts and seeds could provide a person's protein requirements, but legumes and grains were listed in the "bread" group and nuts and seeds in the "fat" group. I decided to take our vegetarian combinations and convert them into filling the "meat" requirement. When I finished writing down recipes and adding up calories, I decided that there might be other diabetics interested in vegetarianism, but who didn't know how to fit this way of eating into their prescribed diet. In this book, I will try to show how easily the diabetic person can lead a vegetarian life and enjoy good health through eating basic nutritious foods. Non-diabetics will also enjoy these recipes, especially weight-conscious diners, because the foods are completely balanced nutritionally and satisfy appetites without the consumption of excess calories.

Patricia M. Mozzer

Being a Vegetarian

There are different kinds of vegetarian diets and different people have different ideas about what it includes. Basically, there are three types: Strict vegetarians or vegans: No animal foods of any kind are eaten. All protein is taken from plant sources. Lacto vegetarians: Animal protein in the form of milk, cheese and other dairy products is included, but not meat, fish, poultry or eggs. Ovo-lacto vegetarians: Animal protein in the form of eggs and dairy products is included, but not meat, fish or poultry.

Unfortunately, much of the nonvegetarian public think vegetarians survive on meals of lettuce and broccoli with a few nuts and seeds. But this is not true. The plant kingdom contains an enormous variety of foods which can be prepared and combined in a great many ways. In general, vegetarians may be more health conscious than the general public, and more concerned with proper nutrition and avoiding processed foods, but this does not mean they are living a deprived existence. The vegetarian diet is an enjoyable diet of much variety.

Throughout history, people have practiced vegetarianism for many reasons. One of the oldest involves the moral question. Some people simply do not believe in killing animals for food. The methods by which animals are raised, slaughtered and marketed are enough reason for them to avoid eating meat.

Other people dislike meat because they think of it as "eating corpses". They feel the sight and smell of dead animals is repulsive, but that a bowl of fruit or a fresh garden vegetable is much more appealing. This feeling for aesthetics is important in defining food choices, not only in vegetarianism, but for example, in a child who refuses to eat his meal because the "peas are touching the mashed potatoes."

Apart from morality and aesthetics, people may become vegetarian for economic and ecological reasons. Growing vegetables is easier on the land and takes less energy to produce and harvest than animals. More food can be grown in less space. Meat production is more costly. Vegetables and grains that are grown to feed cattle and poultry and pigs could be fed directly to people instead.

Other people believe that health is the main advantage to being a vegetarian. In the mid 1800's in this country, a health food movement began. Many reformers were of the Seventh-Day Adventist Church and believed that the body should not be fed an unwholesome diet, meat, alcohol, tobacco or drugs. These people and others believed that meat consumption led to disease and general bad health and that fruits and vegetables had restorative and cleansing powers.

My reasons are a combination of beliefs. There is the acknowledgement that production of vegetables is better for the world ecologically and economically, as well as a life-long preference for vegetables and the belief that since my diet has consisted mainly of vegetables, I have been, in general, healthier and have more energy than before.

The recipes and information in this book are based on ovo-lacto vegetarianism. Dairy products and eggs are included, but not meat, poultry or fish.

Protein, Carbohydrates & Fats

Protein

Our muscles, skin, hair, nails, eyes, teeth, blood, heart, lungs, brain and nerves all contain protein. Protein is also involved in metabolism, which is the process that keeps the body working. Certain essential substances are provided only by protein. All foods contain carbon, oxygen and hydrogen. Only proteins contain nitrogen, sulfur and phosphorus.

Protein is not stored in the body, so a continuous supply is needed. The cells of the body are constantly breaking down and being replaced. Every cell is replaced every 160 days. Certain organs regenerate faster. The liver can regenerate damaged tissue almost immediately.*

When proteins are digested they are broken down into amino acids, the chemical components that make up protein. If calorie intake is adequate the amino acids are used for synthesis of body protein. If either calorie intake is inadequate, protein intake exceeds what is needed by the body or if all the essential amino acids are not present, protein is converted into glucose or fatty acids and used for energy. To use amino acids to the best advantage, there must be a proper proportion of the different kinds of them. There are twenty-two amino acids, but only nine are classified as "essential." The other thirteen are produced by the body if food does not supply them.

*The New Illustrated Medical and Health Encyclopedia, Vol. 3, p.854, H.S. Stuttman Co., Inc., New York, 1975

In the digestive process, the protein is first divided into the amino acids. They are carried by the blood to the liver, from which they are absorbed by the body. They are then recombined to replace worn-out cells, to add to tissues or to make enzymes, hormones or other compounds.

The individual's need for protein is determined by the size, age, health, physical activity and the ability of the person to digest and assimilate the protein taken in. The quality of protein is also a factor here. Meat, fish, poultry, dairy products and eggs contain all of the essential amino acids. They are "complete" sources. Except for soybeans, vegetable sources are "incomplete." They contain varying amounts of different amino acids. By eating two or more vegetable proteins that make up for each other's deficiencies, a complete protein can be created. These complimented vegetable proteins must be eaten at the same meal to get the full value.

Most Americans get more than enough protein. The Food and Nutrition Board of the National Academy of Sciences has established "Recommended Dietary Allowances" (RDA's) for protein for people of different ages and weights. After determining the minimum requirements, the academy added another forty-five percent to the minimum. This means that there is no need to have more than is suggested and that many people can get along with less.

In the following table, determine the grams of protein you should have daily by multiplying the grams of protein per ideal body weight by the age. For example, for a 170 lb. man: 0.36 × 170 = 61.2 grams.

Ages		Grams protein per pound of ideal body weight
0.5	Infants	1.00
0.5-1		0.90
1-3	Children	0.81
4-6		0.68
7-10		0.55
11-14		0.45
15-18		0.39
19 & over	Adults	0.36
Nursing women		0.53
Pregnant women		0.62

*Reprinted from *Jane Brody's Nutrition Book,* by Jane Brody, ©by Jane Brody, used by permission of W W Norton, Inc.

Carbohydrates

Carbohydrates are made up of carbon, hydrogen and oxygen. There are two basic kinds of carbohydrates, the simple carbohydrates, sugars, and the complex carbohydrates, those found in foods as they are directly from the earth, and "refined" or "processed" carbohydrates which are extracted from their natural sources and added to foods. For example, alcohol is a refined substance that the body can use for energy when it is converted to acetate. Packaged cakes, cookies and candy are also refined carbohydrates which are relatively low in nutrients in proportion to the number of calories they contain. This is why they are referred to as "empty" calories.

Carbohydrates provide protein, vitamins, and minerals, and are the only source of the important non-nutrient dietary fiber. Fiber is a carbohydrate from plants which cannot be digested by humans. It supplies no calories, but its "bulk" helps satisfy the appetite and keeps the digestive system in good condition by eliminating wastes regularly. Whole grains, beans, fruits and vegetables are excellent sources of fiber.

Milk and milk products are the only animal foods that contain carbohydrates, all others are from plants. Milk contains the carbohydrate or sugar, lactose. All carbohydrates are made up of one or more sugars. All are broken down by the digestive enzymes and are absorbed into the blood-stream. The liver converts the single molecules into blood sugar or glucose, which is the body's main energy source.

Carbohydrates may be helpful to the diabetic because a diet high in complex carbohydrates helps cut down on the amount of fats the person might eat. This is because most carbohydrates are satisfying and filling. Grains, beans, vegetables and fruits fulfill the physical and psychological need for food. Fruits satisfy a craving for sweetness without an overload of calories, while giving a good amount of nutrients to the body.

In some diabetics, a high carbohydrate diet improves the ability to process blood sugar and may possibly stabilize or lower the insulin requirement. A diet lower in fat and richer in complex carbohydrates and fiber is now recommended more often.

Fats

Dietary fats can be placed into two groups: unsaturated and saturated. Unsaturated (including polyunsaturated and monounsaturated) fats are generally liquid at room temperature and are primarily obtained from vegetable and seed oils. Saturated fats are usually solid at room temperature and are mainly from animal sources; lard, butter, and the fat of muscle meats. Coconut and palm oil are saturated vegetable sources.

Hydrogenated fats are polyunsaturated fats that have been changed to solids or partial solids by the addition of hydrogen, making them saturated. These fats are found in processed foods such as shortening, margarine, some peanut butters, snack foods and some candies.

Some fat is essential to the body. A layer of fat under the skin serves as insulation and conserves body heat. Fat also cushions the vital organs and absorbs shock. It is also a component of every cell membrane and is a supply of reserve energy. Fat is needed to house the fat-soluble vitamins and as a source of essential fatty acids. Of these, linoleic, linolenic, and sometimes arachidonic acids, cannot be made by the body and must be derived from food. Vegetable oils, such as safflower (the highest in linoleic acid), sunflower, corn, soybean, sesame and peanut oil are sources of these essential acids. Only one tablespoon a day of one of these oils is needed to fill the requirement of an adult for fat. The body can make fat from the two other major nutrients, proteins and carbohydrates. If your diet contains more calories than you need for energy each day, then you "get fat."

Fat is digested more slowly than any other nutrient so its presence delays the return of hunger. However, fats also increase the number of calories that a food provides without contributing much of an increase in nutrients, such as French fries instead of a baked or boiled potato (without butter added).

The typical American diet contains much more fat than is needed by the body. The greater the saturated fat intake, the greater the chance of the body building up fat deposits and cholesterol in the blood vessels. Individuals do vary and some people have been found to maintain a low amount of cholesterol in their bodies. But in general, there is evidence that the populations of countries which consume large amounts of saturated fats (the United States and Europe) have a higher rate of heart disease, obesity and diabetes. Mediterranean and Asian countries, in general, have a lower rate. Their diet contains more vegetable oils and fewer animal products.

Minerals

Minerals are inorganic substances that perform many vital functions in the body. Although not as fragile as vitamins, some are water soluble and can be cooked out of foods or bound by substances in the diet that decrease the body's ability to absorb them.

The minerals which are needed by the body can be placed into two categories. Some are needed in relatively large amounts (macrominerals). These are calcium, phosphorus, magnesium, potassium, sodium chloride and sulphur. Trace minerals, those needed in very small amounts, are iron, zinc, selenium, manganese, molybdenum, copper, iodine, chromium, fluorine, silicon, chlorine and cobalt. Except for iron and possibly zinc, a balanced vegetarian diet should provide the proper amounts needed.

Macrominerals

Calcium—Calcium aids in muscle contraction and helps to maintain the delicate acid-alkaline balance in the body. Heart palpitations can be traced to low calcium levels. Calcium must have phosphorus and vitamins A, C and D in order to function. Many sources which provide calcium also contain these other substances needed. For example, bonemeal, an excellent calcium supplement, has the perfect calcium-phosphorus balance built in, and there are other minerals within the bonemeal to facilitate the absorption. Other good vegetarian sources are all dairy and milk products, which contain Vitamin D, green vegetables, which are also good suppliers of vitamins A and C, tofu and cooked beans.

Pregnant women and nursing mothers may need to add about 1 gram (15 grains) of calcium carbonate to their diet each day.
Phosphorus—Phosphorus helps calcium in building bones and teeth. It influences protein, carbohydrate and fat synthesis. It also stimulates muscular contraction, secretion of glandular hormones, nerve impulses and kidney functioning. Phosphorus is the body's energizer.

A deficiency of phosphorus causes weight and appetite loss, nervous disorder, mental sluggishness and general fatigue, although deficiencies of this mineral is rare in the US. Prolonged use of antacids can cause deficiency and interfere with the calcium-phosphorus balance in the body. Good ovo-lacto vegetarian sources of phosphorus are eggs and dairy products. Dried beans and peas also supply phosphorus.

Magnesium—Magnesium is important as an enzyme activator in the manufacture of proteins and the release of energy from muscles, and it also helps in the conduction of nerve impulses to muscles. A deficiency causes muscular twitching and tremors, irregular heartbeat, insomnia, muscle weakness, cramps and shaky hands.

Raw, leafy green vegetables, nuts (mainly almonds and cashews), soybeans, seeds and whole grains are good sources of magnesium.

Potassium—Potassium needs to be in balance with sodium. Together they normalize the heartbeat and central muscle contraction. They also maintain the fluid balance in cells, aid in the transmission of nerve impulses and release energy from carbohydrates, proteins and fats.

Potassium stimulates the kidneys to dispose of body wastes, and the blood also needs a balance of potassium. Deficiencies of this mineral cause constipation, nervous disorder, insomnia, irregular heartbeat and muscle damage.

Good sources of potassium are bananas, citrus fruits, tofu, watercress, green peppers, chicory, blackstrap molasses, figs, dates and avocados.

Sodium—Besides working with potassium, sodium works with chlorine in the blood and lymph system. Its main purpose is to make other blood minerals more soluble and prevent them from becoming clogged or deposited in the blood distribution system.

A sodium deficiency may cause weight loss, stomach and intestinal gas, and muscle shrinkage. Sodium is needed to process amino acids and carbohydrates for digestion. It also helps the formation of saliva, gastric juices and enzymes, and other intestinal secretions.

Good vegetable sources of sodium are beets, carrots, chard and dandelion greens. However, a deficiency of sodium is less of a problem than too much sodium in the form of table salt and salt in many of our processed foods.

Too much salt has been linked to a high blood pressure, heart and kidney disease and stroke. When a person eats something salty, extra water is drawn from the body in an effort to dilute it. Thirst is stimulated and the kidneys are forced to work hard to excrete it. When the body has too much sodium, the kidneys release it into the urine where it is excreted. When sodium is needed, the kidneys reabsorb it and pump it back into the blood. In some people especially sensitive to sodium the kidneys might not be able to excrete enough of the excess. The excess sodium retains water and the volume of blood rises.

The blood vessels become water-logged and more sensitive to nerve stimulation that causes them to contract. The blood has to pass through narrower channels and blood pressure increases. The heart rate is speeded up because there is more blood to pump around the body. Apart from the blood vessels, sodium also increases the amount of water in and around the body tissues, which can cause swelling. If this occurs around the heart, heart failure can occur. Swelling in the legs can interfere with blood returning to the heart and clots may form. Or, swelling around the brain can cause emotional problems, such as irritability or depression. Sodium also draws water and potassium from the cells of the body. Dried out cells don't function properly and can cause you to feel weak and tired.

Enough sodium is naturally present in food and water. Exceptions are those people who exercise strenuously for a long time in hot weather. But even for these people, very little salt is needed to regain the proper balance.

Chloride—Chloride works along with sodium to regulate the balance of body fluids and the acidity and alkalinity balance. It activates the enzyme in saliva and is part of the stomach acid. A deficiency would cause a disturbance in the acid balance of the body, but this is very rare.

Chloride is a component of table salt, so it is also consumed in excess by many people. Enough chloride to supply the body's needs is found in the sources which contain natural sodium.

Sulphur—Sulphur is found in amino-acids and is important in the formation of hair, nails and skin. It helps maintain their smoothness and health. It helps in the blood stream to make the blood more resistant to bacterial infections. It also aids the liver in secreting bile, helps maintain oxygen levels to allow the brain to function properly, and works with B-vitamins that are needed for metabolism and nerve health.

Deficiencies of this mineral are not known in humans. Enough of this mineral is obtained through many foods. The best vegetarian sources are wheat germ, dried beans and peas, and peanuts.

Trace minerals

Iron—Iron's main function is in the formation of hemoglobin in the blood and myoglobin in the muscles, which supply oxygen to the cells. Iron also works with other nutrients to help the respiratory system, and is part of some enzymes and proteins.

A shortage of iron can cause anemia, paleness and poor memory. Good ovo-lacto vegetarian sources are dried beans, egg yolks, green leafy vegetables, molasses and sun-dried raisins. The strongest concentration is found in dried liver.

Zinc—Zinc is a constituent of insulin which is dependent on it for functioning. It also helps manufacture male hormones. It aids in the storage of glycogen, the utilization of carbohydrates and the activation of vitamins. With phosphorus, zinc aids in the respiration process.

A deficiency can cause slow wound healing, and loss of appetite and taste sensation. The best ovo-lacto vegetable sources are eggs, whole grains and milk.

Selenium—Selenium is an antioxidant, which prevents the breaking down of fats and other body chemicals. It interacts with vitamin E.

Deficiencies of selenium are not known in humans. Whole grain cereals, eggs and garlic are the best ovo-lacto vegetable sources.

Manganese—Manganese works with the B-complex vitamins in helping to energize the system. It also helps in building strong bones. It is needed for good enzymatic function in the digestion and utilization of food. Manganese also helps the body resist disease, and promotes good nerve health.

Deficiencies are not known in humans. Blueberries, green leafy vegetables, peas, beets, eggs and whole grains are the best vegetable sources.

Molybdenum—This mineral is part of certain enzymatic processes. Its deficiency is not known in humans. The best vegetable sources are legumes and cereal grains.

Copper—Copper is needed to convert iron into hemoglobin. It also makes tyrosine, an amino acid, and vitamin C into forms usable to the body. A deficiency of copper allows skin sores to develop and not heal, general weakness, and poor respiration. Vegetable sources are almonds, dried beans and peas, whole wheat and prunes.

Iodine—Iodine stimulates the thyroid gland to make the thyroxine hormone which is necessary for metabolism and energy. It also is needed to utilize fat. A deficiency causes slow mental reaction, rapid pulse, heart palpitation, tremor, nervousness, irritability, restlessness and dry hair. The best vegetable sources are vegetables grown in iodine-rich soil, kelp, other seaweeds and onions.

Chromium—Chromium is necessary for the metabolism of glucose. A deficiency may possibly lead to adult-onset diabetes. Whole grains, dried beans, peanuts and brewer's yeast are the best sources.

Fluorine—This mineral helps to prevent tooth decay and to strengthen tooth enamel, but too much can have the opposite effect. Fluoridated water and vegetable foods grown with fluoridated water are the best sources.

Silicon—Silicon is needed for strong bones and teeth. It is part of the cells of the hair, muscles, nails, and connective tissues. A deficiency can cause fatigue, glazed and dull eyes and puffy skin.

The best vegetable sources are buckwheat products, mushrooms, carrots and tomatoes.

Cobalt—Cobalt is a component of vitamin B12. Its sources are mainly of animal origin, but some is found in seaweed.

Vitamins

Vitamins are substances which are are absolutely essential for all the body processes but are needed by the body in small amounts. Vitamins have various functions. They work with enzymes to process fats, carbohydrates, proteins and minerals, and help form blood cells, hormones, genetic material and certain body chemicals. Because vitamins have so many roles, a deficiency of one may affect more than one body function and the lack of different vitamins may produce similar deficiency symptoms.

There are two categories of vitamins: fat soluble and water soluble. Fat soluble vitamins are stored in body fat, so it is not essential to consume them on a daily basis. They need the presence of fat in the diet or bile from the liver to be absorbed. Water soluble vitamins are not stored in the body and must be supplied daily, as they are constantly washed out through urine and perspiration.

Vitamin A—This is a fat-soluble vitamin that is stored in the body, mainly in the liver. Activation of vitamin A depends on having adequate protein. The main functions of this vitamin are to maintain healthy skin, hair and mucous membranes, to aid in the ability to see in dim light, and to promote and maintain bones and teeth development.

Lack of vitamin A can make it difficult for the body to withstand viral infections. The hair and skin can become dry and brittle and the eyes red and itchy.

Vitamin A is easily oxidized (a reaction with oxygen causing spoilage) and needs vitamin E to help prevent this. This vitamin is easily destroyed by light, prolonged heat and rancidity of fats. It is stable in short cooking times so carrots and dark green vegetables should be steamed lightly to obtain the optimum amount of this vitamin.

The best ovo-lacto vegetarian sources of vitamin A are yellow, orange and dark green vegetables, eggs, cheese, fortified butter and dairy products.

Vitamin B Complex—B vitamins are needed for all the living cells of the body to carry out their metabolic processes. The B-complex vitamins are dependent on one another and an inadequate intake of one may affect the utilization of the others. White rice, flour and sugar have had all the B vitamins refined out of them. Mass produced bread products have B vitamins artificially added, but it would be a simpler idea just to leave the wheat unrefined and produce a naturally wholesome bread. B vitamins are also destroyed by intense heat, excessive cooking and light. Baking soda and baking powder also destroy some vitamin B.

These vitamins are responsible for the health of the digestive tract, the skin, mouth, tongue, eyes, nerves, arteries and liver, as well as proper metabolism. Deficiencies cause skin disorders, mental confusion, irritability, muscular weakness and cramps, anemia, smooth tongue, mouth swelling, fatigue, difficulty sleeping, tingling sensations in hands and feet, and depression.

Since vitamin B12 is occurs naturally only in animal products vegetarians who do not use dairy products need to supplement it. Some brands of TVP, tofu, nutritional yeast and tempeh contain added B12. Extra B12 is stored in the liver. A shortage of this essential vitamin can cause severe damage to the nervous system.

Vitamin C—Vitamin C aids in the good health of the body by protecting against colds and building resistance to fatigue and stress. This vitamin is concentrated in the white blood cells, which fight infections. Vitamin C brings hydrogen into the body and helps in proper metabolism. It also helps in absorption of iron, in healing wounds and nurturing bones, skin, teeth and blood vessels. Vitamin C is also a good natural laxative because it dilutes bile which breaks down fat. It is advisable to people who do prolonged hard muscular work, consume chemically fertilized food, or are exposed to air pollution, cigarette smoke, mental stress or infections, to increase their daily vitamin C intake.

A deficiency is marked by weakness, aches, bruising, internal hemorrhaging, bleeding gums, swelling joints and shortness of breath.

The best sources are citrus fruits and juices: orange, grapefruit, lemon, lime and grape. The vegetarian foods most rich in vitamin C are tomatoes, strawberries, melon, green peppers, potatoes, dark green vegetables, and alfalfa.

Like vitamin B, C is water soluble and cannot be stored in the body. This vitamin must be ingested daily. It is sensitive to heat, so vitamin C foods are best eaten raw, or in the case of potatoes, not overcooked. Potatoes should be steamed to avoid contact with water which leaches out the vitamin content. Steaming also cooks vegetables in less time than boiling or baking, and the less time exposed to heat, the better.

Vitamin D—Vitamin D is a fat-soluble vitamin which helps calcium in the formation of bones and teeth. It is necessary for the absorption of calcium and phosphorus. When skin is exposed to the sun, oils in the skin react with the sunlight and synthesize vitamin D.

A prolonged deficiency will cause rickets, a disease which affects children by stunting bone growth and causing malformed teeth and a protruding abdomen. In adults, ostemalasia may result. This is a softening of the bones which can lead to fractures, muscle spasms and twitching.

Sunlight is the most efficient source, other sources being egg yolk and fortified milk.

Vitamin E—This vitamin's main function is to prevent fatty acids from reacting with oxygen and to slow deterioration of the cells. It acts as a natural "preservative." It helps to protect vitamin A, and aids in the formation of red blood cells, muscles and other tissues. It is a fat-soluble vitamin and is stored in the body.

The refining of wheat into white bread, and the heating and hydrogenation of vegetable oil destroys vitamin E. It is possible that the decrease of vitamin E in our bodies since these practices began have caused the increase in heart disease and heart attacks that we know today. This is also due to the buildup of fat deposits in arteries by consuming rich foods. Vitamin E is depleted from the body when called upon to prevent oxidation of fats.

Depletion of this vitamin may cause muscular weakness, oxidized fat deposits and interference with hormone production.

The best sources are vegetable oil, wheat germ and other whole grain cereals and bread, dried beans and green leafy vegetables.

Vitamin K—Vitamin K is a fat-soluble vitamin and needs the presence of bile, which is made by the liver, to be absorbed. It is stable in heat, but is destroyed by light. The main function of this vitamin is to stimulate the production of prothrombin in the blood by the liver. A deficiency will cause blood clotting to take place too slowly.

Enough vitamin K is present in the average diet and it also can be made by the body and the intestines. Impaired fat absorption, liver disease, the prolonged use of antibiotics or sulphur drugs, or an extremely poor diet are the rare causes of deficiency.

The best vegetarian sources of this vitamin are alfalfa, kale, spinach, and cabbage.

A Word on Supplementation

It is important to know that, in general, a diet of adequate quantity and balance probably does not need any supplementation. People who supplement their diets with megadoses of vitamins and minerals can be getting unneccessary or detrimental amounts. It is, however, very hard to achieve the RDA when the food intake is consistently below 1500 calories or when diet variety is limited (in the case of an allergy).

Vegetarian Foods

Grains and Flours

In parts of the world other than the United States, grains provide people with most of their protein. Rice, millet, cracked wheat, barley, buckwheat and corn are the most widely used. These grains, for the most part, are used in an unrefined state. In North America and much of Europe, however, rice and wheat, the most commonly used, are refined into white rice and white flour. This process removes the hull of the grain, along with the bran and the germ. Along with these go most of the protein, calcium, phosphorus, iron, vitamin E and the B vitamins. In the case of white rice, the grain is then polished, coated with a mixture of alcohol and zein (a protein derivative from corn), then treated with calcium and iron salts, dipped into the mix again, and treated with synthetic vitamins. This enrichment does not put back all the nutrients lost in the refining process.

Once you start using brown rice, barley, oats, wheat, millet, and corn you will discover there is more variety in the dishes you prepare with no extra work involved. In cooking grains, the measurement of water to grain need not be exact. Usually a dry amount of grain, 1 cup for example, will need a pot big enough to allow it to triple in volume. Three cups of water to one cup of grain is the basic measurement. (See chart of cooking times on page 46.)

Check bread labels for the words "whole wheat flour". "Wheat" flour means the same as "white" flour in the commercial bread baking world. According to the USDA federal standard, if a bread is said to be "whole wheat", it must be 100% whole wheat.

Commercially baked bread may also contain more than a hundred food and chemical additives. Specialty breads, like rye, pumpernickel, corn or other combinations may contain more white flour than the proper combination of whole flours of which they were traditionally made. For example, pumpernickel, which should be made of a combination of rye and whole wheat flours, may be mainly white, with only 2% rye flour along with caramel coloring and molasses for the pumpernickel appearance.

If you cannot find a suitable whole wheat bread, buy the flour and enjoy the satisfaction of baking your own. Whole wheat flour can be found in any supermarket. Keep it in the refrigerator or in a very cool place to avoid rancidity.

Flour can be made from any grain. Flour and cornmeal can be found in supermarkets, but buckwheat or rice flours are harder to come by. If you really get involved in experimenting with various flours, home grain mills can be purchased through magazine ads (in such magazines as "Country Journal", "Organic Gardening", "Yankee", "Sunset" or other cooking and gardening publications) or possibly at your local appliance store.

One flour you can make in a regular blender is oat flour. Pour 1 cup of rolled oats into the blender or food processor and grind until it is reduced to a powder. This flour absorbs water and can create a heavy bread if used alone, but gives a nice taste variation when mixed partly with whole wheat. It also can be used to make a more nutritious thickener than cornstarch.

Ready-to-Eat Cereals & Crackers

Our favorite cold cereal is simply cold cooked rice, millet, bulghur or barley. If you like a crunchy breakfast but don't know which ready-to-eat cereal is best as far as taste and nutrition, try using plain wheat germ with fruit and yogurt. This offers excellent nutrition with good taste, but no sugar, preservatives or additives. Mix wheat germ with rolled oats, nuts or seeds for variety. Watch out for packaged granola cereals. Even though they may be "all natural," they may be very high in sugar. Wheat flakes, rye flakes, and museli cereals are worth trying, as are any cold cereals made of unprocessed oats, millet, corn, wheat germ, brewer's yeast, seeds, and dries fruit. Avoid cereals with BHT and BHA.

The best rule for buying crackers is the simpler the better. Many crackers are made from only water and whole wheat flour. Try to use crackers without white flour, sugars, artificial color and flavor, citric acid, sodium proprionate, disodium acetate or BHA and BHT. Often, the best crackers may not be in the regular cookie/cracker section, but in the gourmet or dietetic section.

Legumes

Along with grains, legumes are the primary protein source for the vegetarian. Some of the legumes I have listed are more common than others, but all are well worth trying.

Black beans are best in soups. They become very soft in cooking and create a hearty, thick soup.

Black-eyed peas are small and oval shaped. They are white in color with one black "eye." They are popular in Southern and soul food cookery.

Garbanzo beans seem to go weel with every grain. They man be used in main dishes, soups, sandwiches and salads. They are a tan round shaped bean, and take a longer time to cook than most beans except soy.

Great Northern Beans and Navy beans are the beans most of us have eaten as "baked beans." They are also good in soups.

Kidney beans and pinto beans are often used interchangably. Kidney beans are red and kidney shaped. Pintos are beige with dark speckles. They go well with all grains and are good in soups and casseroles.

Lentils can be red, green or brown in color. They are tiny and look much like split peas. They cook in only 30-40 minutes and are excellent in soups and casseroles.

Lima beans are a flat, white bean. You may be more familiar with frozen limas, which are green in color. Dried limas are good for soups and casseroles.

Peanuts are officially legumes, but see them in the "Nut and Seeds" section.

Split peas come in green and yellow. The yellow have a slightly less pronounced flavor. But both (as with lentils), are cooked in the same way. Soup is the traditional use for split peas, but they can be served with a grain or in casseroles.

Soybeans and their products deserve a whole cookbook for themselves. They are the only food in the vegetable kingdom, apart from nutritional yeast, that contains all the essential amino acids, but they still need to eaten with grains to insure that all of the amino acids are present in adequate amounts (see "Combining Proteins", pg. 43). Whole, cooked soybeans can be used in many ways: soups, casseroles, salads, or pureed into a sandwich spread.

Soy grits are toasted pieces of the soy bean. These can be added to casseroles, or put into bread to give it a chopped nut effect with fewer calories and lower fat.

Tofu, a versatile soybean product,is a solid white cake of bean curd, made in a way that is similar to the cheese-making process. Tofu has a smooth texture and mold flavor which blends well with any food. It needs no cooking which makes it good for fast meals, salads and sandwiches.

Tempeh is a high protein food made from soybeans by a natural culturing process. It contains more riboflavin, niacin and B6 than regular soybeans. It is low in calories and cholesterol free. The flavor of tempeh depends on what bean or bean and grain or nut combination it is made from. Most tempeh in this country is made from soybeans. It's available at health food stores. Tempeh is the most digestible form of soybeans. Keep tempeh refrigerated and steam for 10 minutes before using. It can be diced or grated to add protein, vitamins and minerals to salads, sandwiches, soups and casseroles. Marinating in herbs, spices or tamari can vary the flavor of tempeh as you combine it with grains and vegetables.

Soy flour is a heavy flour which can make your homemade baked goods contain complete protein. This flour should never be eaten raw, only in thoroughly cooked dishes or baked goods. It has a strong, nutty taste. Use ¼ cup to each 1 cup of whole wheat flour to complement protein.

Texturized vegetable protein (TVP) is made from defatted soy flour. The soy flour has the oil extracted from it and what remains is mostly protein and carbohydrate. The defatted soy flour is cooked under pressure and extruded through holes, then cut into chunks. This dry precooked food and then be hydrated and cooked into many dishes.

Tamari is a type of soy-sauce. It is naturally aged and contains no chemical colorings, as many soy sauces do. It is high in sodium, however, and should be used sparingly.

Legumes are readily available in supermarkets. Soybean products, such as tofu and tempeh are becoming more common in many markets also, but in some areas, you may still have to find a natural food store or co-op to obtain them.

Nuts and Seeds

Nuts and seeds follow legumes in their ability to supply protein. Actually, they are as rich in protein and some have a higher NPU (see Glossary), but people tend to eat fewer nuts, as they are more filling and high in calories.

Seeds are better than nuts when it comes to usable protein. Sunflower seeds are best, since they supply good quality protein and are an important source of Vitamin B6. They also are lower in calories per gram of usable protein than sesame seeds or nuts.

Nuts are sold shelled and unshelled, except for cashews which are never in a shell. Unshelled nuts have the advantage of the shell as a guard against nutritional loss and chemical contamination. Unshelled nuts are treated with lye and gas to soften and loosen them and the shells are usually bleached and may be colored or waxed. Use pistachios that haven't been dyed red. When buying unshelled nuts, be sure they have no mold and have a minimum of shell damage.

Nuts in the shell are unroasted, except for peanuts. Shelled nuts, however, may be raw or roasted. They may be whole or in pieces. Almonds are blanched by means of a hot-water bath to remove the outer skin. This is merely for cosmetic preference. Unblanched almonds are also available and contain more nutrients.

Avoid buying unshelled nuts that have been roasted in oil and salted. These have too much additional fat roasted into them.

Nuts and seeds must be protected from heat, air and moisture. They should be stored, shelled or unshelled in a covered container in a cool place. In hot weather, keep them in the refrigerator.

Nuts and seeds are a good addition to any vegetarian meal. Use them in main dishes, breakfast cereals, pancakes, baked products, salads, sandwiches, vegetable stir-fry dishes, and many other ways. Any nuts or seeds can be ground into peanut butter consistency. If you want to do this at home, be sure to keep track of the amount of nuts and the amount of oil you use. Basically, 2 cups of nuts, ground into a powder, with ¼ cup of safflower oil slowly added is a good measurement. One tablespoon of most nut butters can be counted the same as peanut butter (1 high fat meat exchange or 1 lean meat exchange plus 1 fat exchange).

As for peanut butter, buy brands which are made only from peanuts. Avoid brands with sugars, hydrogenated shortening and, preferably, salt. You may not be able to get salt-free brands in a supermarket, but most natural food stores have them. It is better to add a small amount of salt yourself, if you are trying to use less, but haven't gotten away from it completely.

Vegetables

Grains, legumes, nuts and seeds are important protein sources, as well as minerals, vitamin B complex and E, but vegetables are needed to round out these vitamin and mineral requirements. Except for vitamin D, every vegetable is strong in one or more of the essential vitamins and minerals. A good variety of them is needed to cover all the nutrients. The nutritional value of vegetables varies with the kind of vegetable, the season of harvesting, soil, storage and preparation. In general, certain vegetables can be counted on for certain nutrients. All yellow, orange and dark green vegetables are rich in Vitamin A. Green leafy vegetables supply, in addition to A, Vitamin C, iron, riboflavin and calcium. When fresh, most vegetables are reliable vitamin C sources, especially when eaten raw.

Sprouts are easy to grow and are a good source of protein, vitamin C and trace minerals. By growing sprouts, you can always have a fresh vegetable to add to soups, sandwiches, and salads. See page 72 for directions for making them.

In most cases, vegetables are at their best nutritionally if they are eaten soon after harvesting. Of course, this isn't always possible. Nutritional losses occur due to chemical changes within the plant. These can be speeded up by heat or slowed down by cold.

Packaged frozen vegetables go from the field to the freezing and packing plant. They may be frozen immediately, or they may be waiting around losing vitamins for a few days before they are processed. The consumer has no way of knowing. In addition, these vegetables may be sprayed with chemicals to avoid spoilage while they are waiting to be frozen. Before they are frozen, they are blanched with hot water to destroy certain enzymes which cause spoilage during storage. This process does kill some vitamin C and there is additional vitamin loss in the blanching process. When frozen vegetables arrive at the supermarket there is no way to know how long they have been in the freezer case, and even when taken home, they may not be used for another week or more. Although freezing has slowed down much of the nutritional losses, the older the vegetables become, the greater the loss. If the vegetables have become partially defrosted through mishandling at any point in the process, further spoilage occurs.

With all those chances for nutritional loss, freezing is still better than canning. The heat involved in canning changes the color, flavor and texture of the vegetables (or fruit). It also kills much of the vitamin content. Much of these nutrients are lost in the water in which the vegetables are canned, as most people usually throw this salty liquid out. Canned vegetables are also subjected to the addition of acids to ensure the retardation of bacterial growth. Acids (usually baking soda) destroy B vitamins. Salt, sugar, artificial coloring and flavoring, and other additives may also be used in the processing.

Fresh vegetables, ideally, are the best. Still, it may not be known how fresh they are or if they have been sprayed. Locally grown produce is your best bet. Often, foods that are grown locally will be thus advertised. Try to fit those into your meals when you can get them. If you are lucky enough to live in a section of the country where there is always some variety of vegetable in season, concentrate on using whatever it is. If you live in a northern area, have plenty of squash, green beans, tomatoes, etc., all summer and forget frozen vegetables until the fresh ones in the markets begin to look like they've been on a long, slow train. Be sure to wash all fresh vegetables well. Do not soak them, but scrub them in cold, soapy water. Soaps can remove some chemicals that plain water cannot. Rinse them well. Select vegetables that look fresh and have no bruises, handle them carefully and buy only what you need. Plan to eat them within one or two days. Root vegetables; potatoes, carrots, parsnips, onions, turnips; can be kept longer, but they still suffer nutritional loss too.

Vegetables should be peeled only when the skin is unpalatable, such as turnips, rutabagas, or the tough stem ends of broccoli. Cook yams, squash and potatoes in their jackets. Peel them when cooked or eat the peel too. (Yes, even butternut or acorn squash.)

Steaming is my favorite method for cooking vegetables as it is easy, fast, and there is no contact with water. This minimizes nutrient loss. Steaming also helps to reduce the loss of the bright color of the vegetable. Broccoli retains its bright green and winter squash its bright orange, whereas boiling creates a dull, soggy, tasteless product. Steaming also retains flavor, thus reducing the desire to add salt to the vegetable.

Pressure cooking is also an excellent method. Timing must be accurate, or the vegetables can quickly become overcooked. The greatest percentage of vitamins is saved using this method.

Cooking times for steaming or pressure cooking vary from vegetable to vegetables. Also, the same vegetable can be different, one bunch of broccoli may be tougher than another or the green beans bought this shopping trip may be larger than last week's. Experiment and cook until the vegetable is just tender, not mushy. When steaming vegetables, you will find that if you turn off the heat when they are half done, they will keep cooking if kept tightly covered. Frozen vegetables need little more than to be heated thoroughly by the steam, as they have already been blanched. .

The best tips to remember for vegetables are to buy fresh, seasonal vegetables first; fresh, good-looking vegetables that are in their peak season wherever they came from, second; frozen vegetables third; and canned vegetables least often. Organically grown vegetables have had no chemicals used in their production.

Fruits

Fruit provides the body with natural sugar to satisfy the sweet craving. Adding fruit to your daily diet also helps to fill much of the vitamin and mineral requirements. Most fruits contain varying amounts of vitamins A and C, potassium and some calcium and iron.

As with vegetables, the best fruit you can get is that which is in season and grown locally. Fruits are usually grown in chemically fertilized soil. Fruit trees and bushes are sprayed with herbicides and pesticides, unless they are organic. Some fruits have a protective outer layer which is never eaten. The edible part is thus protected from surface spraying. Examples include pineapples, bananas and melon. Apples, pears, peaches and other fruits that have no protection, should be scrubbed thoroughly before eating. Grapes, in particular, are heavily sprayed, and need to be thoroughly washed.

Fruits are often waxed or colored to make them look more appealing and fresher. Oranges growing on trees are not bright orange and neither are lemons such a bright yellow. Grating these rinds into your cooking ingredients may be adding some dangerous dyes into your food.

With waxed apples or pears, or any extremely shiny fruit, not much can be done but to peel them. Many vitamins reside in the peel, but the wax is almost impossible to remove.

Unfortunately, many fruits are picked when immature and never ripen sufficiently. They may become dried out and tasteless, instead of juicy and sweet.

Pick fruit that has good color naturally, such as firm red or green apples with no bruises and preferably unwaxed. Bananas should be partially green and have few surface bruises. Wait until their jackets are a mellow yellow with a few brown speckles before eating. This is the peak of their ripeness. When buying berries, do not buy light colored ones (immature), or ones that look over ripe. They should be plump and firm. When buying citrus, pick fruits that feel heavy for their size. Thin-skinned citrus are juicier. Avoid ones that yield to pressure (true of any fruit). If available, buy uncolored citrus. Peaches, nectarines and plums should be rich in color. They should be dark purple or solid yellow with bright orange and they should be firm and heavy. Melons are often difficult fruits to judge for ripeness. Look for ones with even color and with a slight softening at the blossom end.

Fruits should be stored in the refrigerator unless they need a day or two to ripen. Bananas can be refrigerated when ripe, however, their jackets will soon turn brown. This does not mean they have rotted inside.

Fortunately, fruits have a higher natural acid content than vegetables, so loose fewer vitamins in the canning process. The peeling, cutting and heating of the canning process does decrease some of the nutrients, and, as with vegetables, most of these nutrients are lost if the canning water is thrown out.

Fruits are rich in natural sugars, but manufacturers add sugar to canned fruits to maintain the texture and as a preservative. It is possible to buy only lightly sweetened fruit, or fruit preserved in its own juice. The label must state if sugar is added, so read the label.

Frozen fruits may also have sugar added, particularly frozen berries. They may have other colorings, salt or acids added. It is best to choose the fresh seasonal fruits and avoid canned or frozen ones.

Diabetics are often warned to stay away from dried fruit because these are such a concentrated source of sugar. It is true that only 3 prunes, 1½ figs, or 2 tablespoons of raisins equal one fruit exchange. Yet, it is possible to enjoy these fruits in these amounts because of the concentrated flavor that can add much taste to a dish of oatmeal or a cup of yogurt. Use them in the amounts suggested for one serving, and they will give you a naturally sweet treat with all the iron and nutrients of fresh fruit. The drying process is such that the vitamins and minerals are retained.

If possible, get sun-dried and not artificially dehydrated fruit. This latter method uses sulphur dioxide. This is always stated on the label (some sun-dried fruits contain it too). Other ingredients to avoid are added sugar, corn syrup or honey, and preservatives.

Eggs

Eggs are a good source of many vitamins and minerals and are high in protein. They are low in saturated fat, but are high in cholesterol. Unfortunately, they are often cooked with bacon grease or butter or served with buttery toast, bacon or sausage which increases both saturated fat and cholesterol levels. By reducing or eliminating those fats, eggs can be a healthy food. This is not to advocate unlimited use of eggs in your diet, but only to say that as a food used in the ovo-lacto vegetarian diet, it does have much to offer, both nutritionally and in creating a tasteful diet.

With all that the egg has going for it, it is unfortunate that modern egg production methods have done so much to contaminate it. Laying hens are usually given antibiotics and chemicals in their feed. These are transferred to the egg. Try to find eggs that have come from "free-running" chickens, that is, chickens which have been allowed outside and have been fed grain rather than chemical formulas. These eggs are often more flavorful too.

One advantage in buying eggs is that most are fresh and some of the containers may be dated. Make sure that there are no cracked eggs in the carton. Brown and white eggs are the same nutritionally. Eggs are graded for quality and size. U.S. Grade AA Fancy Fresh is the best. Small, medium, large or extra large are the sizes and do not relate to the quality.

I do not advocate the use of liquid eggs, frozen, dried or other egg substitutes. There may be unnecessary chemicals added, and, depending on the process, they may be less than nutritionally adequate.

Don't wash eggs, as this cuts down on the egg's natural germ protection coating. Eggs can be kept well for several weeks in the refrigerator.

Milk and Milk Products

Milk is an important food. It is an excellent source of protein, calcium and phosphorus, and is usually supplemented with vitamins A and D.

As an ovo-lacto vegetarian, I do use some milk, but this is usually in baked products or on breakfast cereals or blended breakfast milkshakes. Because of the milkfat in whole milk products, it is preferable to use only low-fat, skim or non-fat dry milk. As a change from milk, try plain yogurt or kefir. Buttermilk is produced with much altering of the natural product. It is often made from stale, reclaimed pasteurized milk, and rarely comes from the liquid that remains after butter is churned, as it did years ago.

Yogurt is produced from the interaction of milk with certain bacterial cultures. All the nutrition of milk is contained in the yogurt. Many people who cannot digest regular milk can digest yogurt. Yogurt culture is also important as a cleanser in the intestine, as it is able to destroy many harmful bacteria.

Kefir has all the benefits of milk and yogurt. Like yogurt, it contains bacterial cultures. In fact, it tastes rather like yogurt, but is of a thinner consistency.

Both kefir and yogurt are available plain or with sweetener and fruit. Buy only the plain and add your own fruit. The flavored yogurts and kefir contain sugar. Avoid brands that include sugar, honey, modified food starch, sodium citrate, gelatin, corn syrup, artificial color and flavor, citric acid, tartaric acid or potassium sorbate. Yogurt can be found in most supermarkets, but kefir may be harder to find. Natural food stores may be the more likely source. (Yogurt is easy to make; see the recipe on page 129).

Along with whole milk, there are a number of other milk products that should be avoided. Cream, whipped cream, half and half and sour cream contain too much saturated fat. Imitation cream, imitation milk and non-dairy products are chemical substances which may also be high in saturated fat, as they are often made of coconut or palm oil. They usually also contain chemical stabilizers, emulsifiers, corn syrup and artificial flavorings. If you feel you must occasionally use some cream, use the real thing, dairy cream.

Evaporated and sweetened condensed milk usually have chemicals added to maintain uniform taste and texture. Sweetened condensed milk also contains some form of sugar.

Cheese

Cheese is an excellent, concentrated source of many of the nutrients contained in milk. In the ovo-lacto vegetarian diet, cheese can be used to increase the protein quality of grains, nuts and seeds, or beans. However, many cheeses are high in saturated fats and those should used in moderation. There are many kinds of cheeses and many cheese-making processes, which can affect the protein quality and fat content of the product. It's good to be aware of which cheeses are best nutritionally.

Cheese making can be divided into two categories, natural and processed. Natural cheeses are made from milk solids by separating curds and whey, heating, stirring and pressing into final form. Cow's or goat's milk may be used, and it may be from whole milk or skim milk, cream and/or whey. Salt is added to most cheeses.

Unfortunately, coloring, preservatives, acidifying agents or other additives may become part of the ingredients. These may not always appear on the label. Usually, imported cheeses have no additives, but I don't mean to warn you away from all American made cheeses. Feta cheese, for example, from whatever country, is chemical free. Mozzarella, also, is usually a safe choice.

Edam cheese, from the Netherlands, is made with partially skim milk, so is a good choice as a low-fat cheese. Provolone, from Italy and the United States, contain unstated coloring additives, but the preservatives are always on the label.

You might consider substituting gruyere for Swiss. The milk used in Swiss cheese may be bleached to give it a paler yellow color. This reduces the vitamin A content. Mold inhibitors, and preservatives may or may not be added and may or may not be on the label. Gruyere is never colored or bleached, and any additives are always stated.

Among the cheddar cheeses, Vermont is a good choice. Orange cheddar cheese contains food coloring so you may prefer to use yellow varieties.

Other cheeses which are largely unadulterated are all of the Danish cheeses, roquefort and gouda.

Cottage cheese is made from skim milk. "Creamed" cottage cheese means cream has been added, and along with it, many additives are possible. Look for brands that don't contain acids, vegetable gums, stabilizers or artificial flavoring. Opt for those that are low fat or uncreamed and try out unsalted brands.

Ricotta cheese is a good cheese to use because you always know what you're getting. As with cottage cheese, the additives are stated on the label, and you can get whole milk or skimmed milk brands.

Cream cheese is a high fat, low protein product which should be used infrequently. Avoid any brands with additives or try neufchatel cheese which is very similar, but lower in fat.

Processed cheeses are are heated to stop the natural cheese ripening process. This, with the addition of emulsifiers and stabilizers, creates a smooth texture and consistent flavor. This makes for an easy melting, easy spreading product, but the dull texture and flavor, and the numerous additives make it a poor choice. Cheeses under this category are known as pasteurized process cheese, pasteurized process cheese food, pasteurized process cheese spread, cold pack cheese, smoked cheese and blended cheese.

Pasteurized process cheese is made by grinding and blending one or more natural cheeses, then heating and mixing with water and emulsifier. The emulsifier (which is various amounts and combinations of thirteen different chemicals), artificial coloring, artificial flavoring and preservatives give this cheese its smooth texture. American Cheese and Pasteurized Process Swiss are examples.

Pasteurized Process Cheese Food is similar to the pasteurized process cheese, but it contains less cheese and more water. It is lower in fat, but high in chemicals. American cheese is available in this form also.

Pasteurized Process Cheese Spread has even more water added, and needs chemical stabilizers to prevent the separation of the ingredients. This comes packed in jars.

Cold pack cheeses do not undergo heating in the processing, but may have sugar or corn syrup added.

Smoked cheeses are usually "smoked" through the burning of sawdust. The hydrocarbons in wood smoke are suspected carcinogens. Along with the already chemical-filled processed cheese, the hydrocarbons make this food one to avoid.

Choose a natural rather than a processed cheeses. Remember, the word "American" is a clue to determining a processed cheese.

Butter and Margarine

Substituting margarine for butter because it is lower in fat or calories is a misconception. The fat content of both butter and margarine is 80%. Margarine's fat may be from animal fat, vegetable oil, or a combination of the two. Margarines with animal fat are no better than butter if saturated or unsaturated fat is the main concern. Vegetable oil margarines are made from polyunsaturated oils, but the process which turns them into margarines is at least a partial hydrogenating process. This creates a saturated fat from a previously unsaturated one. If the label states that the fat is "hydrogenated or hardened oil," like partially hardened safflower oil, there are more unsaturated fats. Because of the confusion and variety of margarines, some vegetarians prefer to use butter, which has less additives, colorings, preservatives and refinement than margarine.

When buying butter, buy unsalted, and if stated, uncolored brands. Although I recommend butter as preferable to margarine, I also recommend using a minimum of it. Spread your bread with nut butters, tahini, oil, cottage or ricotta cheese or homemade dressings.

Mayonnaise, Oil, and Salad Dressings

Bottled salad dressings have an amazingly long list of ingredients for a product that should be a simple blend of oil, vinegar and herbs or spices. Along with these, salt, sugar, MSG, stabilizers, emulsifiers, preservatives, coloring and starches may be used. Also, many brands use strong, cheap white vinegar and cottonseed oil, which comes from a heavily sprayed crop, It is safer to make your own dressings (see recipes).

Mayonnaise can contain many undesirable ingredients, such as sugars, starch and preservatives. Check the label and buy the purest possible brand.

When buying oil, you will find that the most common product is "pure vegetable oil." This is no assurance of purity. Fortunately, the kinds of oils used are stated on the label. Look for brands that don't contain cottonseed oil, as it is heavily sprayed because cotton's main use is not as a food crop. Also avoid oils with preservatives such as BHA, BHT, citric acid and polysorbate 80.

Corn, canola and safflower oil are excellent sources of polyunsaturates. Try to get these in brands without additives. Peanut and soybean oil are other good sources and brands without chemicals can be found. Olive oil is the only oil that is always unrefined and without additives. It is cold-pressed, which means it is removed from the plant by pressing, instead of by heating or by means of a solvent. Heat and solvents destroy vitamin E, which is a natural antioxidant. This is why refined oils can become rancid and manufacturers add chemicals to slow this process. However, if you buy refined, unpreserved oils and use them within a month or two, no rancidity should occur, especially if kept in the refrigerator.

Honey and Molasses

In my recipes, I occasionally use blackstrap molasses or honey in small amounts. I feel that this is better than using chemical sugar substitutes or white sugar.

When sugarcane goes through processing to yield white sugar, the residue is blackstrap molasses. This contains all the nutrients of the original sugar cane, which are B vitamins, calcium, phosphorus and iron. This has a strong, almost bitter taste and very little is needed in a recipe. Unsulphured molasses also contains the same nutrients as blackstrap, but has a more mellow taste. It is not a by-product of sugar refining, but rather is manufactured for the molasses itself.

Honey, the nectar of flowers, converted to a rich syrup by bees, is another sugar substitute to be used in small amounts. All honey, fortunately, is fairly free of pesticide residues because bees are sensitive to them and would not live long enough to produce honey. You may prefer to buy unfiltered, raw honey. This honey has not been subjected to heat and so contains traces of nutrients and enzymes. Because honey may contain botulism spores, health professionals warn against feeding it to infants under one year of age, as they can be especially sensitive to those spores. Raw honey (and unsulphured molasses) can be found in super-markets. Blackstrap molasses may be found in natural food stores or co-ops.

Tomato Sauce

Buy only the brands of tomato sauce which do not contain artificial color, artificial flavor, preservatives, starchy thickeners, corn syrup, sugar, or salt. It is better to add a small amount of salt yourself if you must. In my recipes, I use only a small amount of tomato sauce, preferring to use more vegetables along with the sauce for a more interesting flavor. It is a good low-fat alternative to cream or cheese sauces but if you're not careful, tomato sauce calories can add up quickly. It's best to use it as a flavoring rather than the traditional way of pouring it over the bowl of pasta or whatever dish you are preparing.

Nutritional and Brewer's Yeast

Nutritional yeast (saccharomyces cerevisiae) grown in a molasses solution has a good flavor (somewhat like cheese) and has B vitamins and good quality protein. Children like it sprinkled on pasta, rice, other grains, beans, popcorn and vegetables. It is easily digestible and contains all the essential amino acids. Riboflavin content gives it a yellow color. Added to soups and gravies it has a nutty flavor.

This yeast comes in both flakes and powder and is available at health food stores. Not more than 3 tsp. of powder or 4 tsp. of flakes should be eaten per person per day. Check the label of the yeast you buy to see if it has vitamin B12. This important vitamin is the most likely to be deficient in a total vegetarian diet. The inclusion of good tasting nutritional yeast daily will help supply B12.

Brewer's yeast is a by-product of the beer-making process. There are other yeast products, such as torula, which are grown in laboratories, (but still unnaturally) and which contain the same nutrients. These yeast products are an excellent source of the B-vitamin complex and are a source of complete protein. These products can be found in any natural food store or co-op, or in many supermarkets. Yeast is also available in pill form as a food supplement.

Try using nutritional yeast in casseroles, sprinkled on cereals or in blended drinks. Yeast can taste different when mixed with different foods, but always lends an interesting flavor that is worth experimenting with.

Yeast is also a source of the trace mineral chromium, which has been studied as a possible aid in the treatment of adult-onset diabetes. Chromium seems to enhance the insulin production of the pancreas. It is believed that a deficiency of this mineral may be a factor in the development of diabetes.

Kelp

Kelp is the general name for various large, brown seaweeds which are rich in iodine and other minerals. It is a good addition to a low-salt diet because it provides iodine without the sodium. It is available in tablets or powder in natural food stores and some drug stores. It is preferable to use the powder, as the tablets, by law, can contain only 0.15 milligrams of iodine. Try kelp by adding it to any casserole, salad dressing or soup.

Coffee and Tea

There are many brands and flavors of herbal teas on the market today. Take a break from regular coffee and tea to experiment with this wide variety. Most of these teas do not contain caffeine. Because of this, you may find that they soothe your nerves after a long day much better than black teas or coffee.

The caffeine in tea and coffee can have a variety of effects on the body. It is a stimulant, which helps you to wake up in the morning or to pick you up late in the day. It has a direct stimulating effect on the parts of the brain which are concerned with thoughts, heart rate, respiration and muscle coordination. It can raise the basal metabolic rate and so increase the number of calories burned, but it also ignites the release of insulin, causing blood sugar to drop.

The positive effect of caffeine is that it stimulates blood flow to the heart by dilating the coronary arteries. It also constricts the blood vessels which go to the brain and so is included in some headache remedies, since dilated blood vessels contribute to headaches.

There are more potential hazards than good points about caffeine however. Caffeine is an addictive substance, and for all it can do to relieve headaches, it can addict you to the remedy. Excessive caffeine can produce an abnormally fast heart beat and also increase blood pressure. It also is linked to ulcers and other digestive problems. Heartburn is at many times the result of too much coffee or tea. Anxiety and muscular jitteriness are other problems caused by too much caffeine.

Along with caffeine, the tannic acid in tea, the dyes used in the black or orange pekoe leaves and the chemicals in the tea bags are also health concerns. Try to reduce or eliminate coffee and tea in your diet. If you still wish to drink it, try brewing the tea for a shorter time and don't let perked coffee stand with the coffee grounds. Reduce your consumption to two or three cups a day. Do not use any artificial sweeteners, sugar or honey (unless you count the calories of the sugar or honey).

Leavening Agents

Baking soda, baking powder, yeast and eggs can be considered leavening agents. Baking soda works by releasing carbon dioxide as the result of mixing it with a liquid ingredient such as milk or water. Baking powder is made of baking soda, an acid salt to produce a more controlled leavening action, and a starch to prevent the powder from caking. Yeast works by giving off carbon dioxide as the result of fermentation. This begins when the yeast is mixed with a warm liquid. The white of eggs can be a leavening agent too. They can be beaten until stiff peaks form and then can be folded into the batter.

Yeast is the best leavening agent. It contains B vitamins and destroys none of the nutrients in the baked product. Egg whites create a leavened, but heavier product, but you may find that the texture is pleasant and satisfying. Unfortunately, baking soda and baking powder, which may seem the easiest to use, affect the nutrient thiamine in the flour. Some of the B vitamins are destroyed. There is also concern that aluminum-based baking powders are carcinogenic. Use baking powder that does not contain aluminum, but uses tartar or phosphate in the ingredients. The use of whole wheat flour and wheat germ with their higher amounts of B vitamins than bleached flour, is especially important if these baking powders are to be used.

The Exchange System

The exchange system is a plan in which all foods are placed into categories according to whether they consist mainly of fats, carbohydrates or protein. This method helps the diabetic person to keep the balance between calories and insulin and to assure a balanced diet. There are six groups. They are: (1) the milk group; (2) the vegetable group; (3) the fruit group; (4) the starchy vegetable/bread group; (5) the meat group; and (6) the fats group.

The amount of exchanges for each of the six categories that a person requires depends on weight, age, activity and method of treatment of the diabetes. It is most important for an insulin dependent diabetic to stay on a regulated diet to avoid hypoglycemia and hyperglycemia. Because the insulin is injected, it will go to work no matter how much or how little food is eaten. A diabetic on oral medication should be aware also of calories and proper eating habits to possibly improve or even eliminate the disease. Since most of these people's bodies still produce insulin, correct diet can make a big difference in well-being.

The following pages present the six food groups, many of the foods representing the group, and the calories, fat, carbohydrate and protein amounts of one exchange unit of food. This is the 'traditional' diabetic system and includes a meat list. The next section will combine many of the foods within the starchy vegetable/bread group to achieve the protein provided by the meat group.

Group one is the bread, cereal and starchy vegetable group. One exchange equals 15 grams of carbohydrate, 3 grams of protein and 80 calories. This list shows the measurement of each of the foods in this group to equal one exchange:

Bread:
White	1 slice
Whole Wheat	1 slice
Rye or Pumpernickel	1 slice
Raisin	1 slice
Bagel	½
English Muffin	½
Plain Roll	1 small
Hot Dog Roll	½
Hamburger Bun	½
Dried Bread Crumbs	3 Tbsp.
Tortilla, 6" dia.	1

Crackers:
Graham (2½" sq.)	3
Rye crisp, 2" × 3½"	4
Saltines	6

Legumes
Dried beans, peas, lentils (cooked)	⅓ cup

Cereal:
Bran Flakes	½ cup
Other ready-to-eat unsweetened cereal	¾ cup
Puffed Wheat	1½ cup

(cont.)

(Cont.)

		Starchy Vegetables:	
Cereal (cooked)	½ cup	Corn	½ cup
Rice (cooked)	⅓ cup	Corn on cob, 6″	1
Pasta (cooked)	½ cup	Lima Beans	½ cup
Popcorn, popped,		Peas (green)	½ cup
unbuttered	3 cups	Potato, white	1 small
Cornmeal (dry)	2½ Tbsp	Potato, mashed	½ cup
Flour, whole wheat		Squash, winter,	
unbleached	2½ Tbsp	acorn or butternut	¾ cup
Wheat germ	3 Tbsp.	Yam or sweet potato	⅓ cup

Group two is the meat group. One meat exchange equals 7 grams of protein. Lean meats have 3 gms. fat and 55 calories; medium-fat meats, 5 gms. fat and 75 calories; high-fat meats, 8 gms. fat and 100 calories. The following amounts for each food in this group equals one exchange.

Lean Meats and Substitutes:

Lean Beef, Lean Pork	1 oz.
Chicken, Turkey	1 oz.
All fresh and frozen fish	1 oz.
Crab, Lobster, Shrimp, Clams	2 oz.
Tuna, water packed	¼ cup
Oysters	6 medium
Sardines	2 medium
Cottage Cheese	¼ cup
Grated parmesan	2 Tbsp.

Medium-Fat Meats and Substitutes

Most Beef, Pork, Lamb, Veal	1 oz.
Eggs	1
Poultry with skin	1 oz.
Canned Salmon and Tuna with oil	¼ cup
Ricotta	¼ cup
Mozzarella Cheese	1 oz.
Tofu	4 oz.

High-Fat Meats and Substitutes

Most Prime Beef, Spareribs	1 oz.
Fried Fish	1 oz.
Cheddar, Swiss, etc.	1 oz.
Hot Dog	1 medium
Peanut Butter	1 Tbsp.

Group three is the vegetable exchange group. One exchange equals about 5 grams of carbohydrate, 2 grams of protein and 25 calories. Either one-half cup cooked or one cup raw of the following vegetables equals one exchange, unless specified below.

Asparagus Beans	Dandelion
(green, wax, Italian)	Kale
Bean	Mustard
Sprouts	Turnips
Beets	Kohlrabi
Broccoli	Leeks
Brussels	Mushrooms, cooked
Sprouts	Okra
Cabbage,cooked	Onions
Carrots	Pea pods
Cauliflower	Rutabaga
Celery	Sauerkraut
Eggplant	Spinach, cooked
Green	Summer Squash
Pepper	Tomatoes, one
Greens:	Tomato Juice
Beets	Turnips
Chard	Water chestnuts
Collards	Zucchini, cooked

These raw vegetables may either be used freely or as a one cup serving as indicated:

Cucumber, 1 cup	Lettuce
Chicory	Parsley
Chinese Cabbage, 1 cup	Radishes, 1 cup
Endive	Spinach
Escarole	Watercress

Group four is the fruit list. One exchange of fruit equals 15 grams of carbohydrate and 60 calories. This list shows the amounts of fruits to use for one exchange:

Apple	1 medium	Berries:	
Apple Juice	1/2 cup	Blackberries	3/4 cup
Applesauce	1/2 cup	Blueberries	3/4 cup
Apricots (fresh)	4 medium	Raspberries	1 cup
Apricots (dried)	4 halves	Strawberries	1 1/4 cup
Banana	1/2 large	Cherries	12 large
			(cont.)

(Cont.)

Cider	½ cup	Nectarine	1
Cranberry Juice	⅓ cup	Orange Juice	½ cup
Dates	2 ½	Papaya	1 cup
Figs (fresh)	1 ½	Peach	1
Figs (dried)	1 ½	Pear	1 small
Grapefruit	½	Persimmon (native)	2 medium
Grapes	15	Pineapple, fresh	¾ cup
Grape Juice	⅓ cup	Pineapple Juice	½ cup
Mango	½ small	Plums	2 medium
Melon:		Prunes	3 medium
Cantaloupe	⅓ small	Prune Juice	⅓ cup
Honeydew	medium	Tangerine	2 medium
Watermelon	1¼ cup		

The fifth group in the exchange system is the milk group. One exchange equals 12 grams of carbohydrate, 8 grams of protein and 90 calories (based on skim milk). This list shows the kinds and amounts of milk or milk products to use for one milk exchange.

Non-Fat Fortified Milk

Skim or non-fat milk	1 cup
Powdered non-fat dry measure	⅓ cup
Canned, evaporated skim milk	½ cup
Buttermilk made from skim milk	1 cup
Yogurt made from skim milk (plain, unflavored)	1 cup

Low-Fat Fortified Milk

1% fat fortified milk (omit ½ fat exchange)	1 cup
2% fat fortified milk (omit 1 fat exchange)	1 cup
Yogurt made from 2% fortified milk (plain, unflavored) (omit 1 fat exchange)	1 cup

Whole Milk (omit 2 fat exchanges)

Whole milk	1 cup
Canned, evaporated whole milk	½ cup
Buttermilk made from whole milk	1 cup
Yogurt made from whole milk (plain, unflavored)	1 cup
Kefir made from whole milk	1 cup

Group six contains the fat exchanges. One exchange equals 5 grams of fat and 45 calories. Each measurement of the foods below equal one exchange.

Unsaturated Fats

Margarine, oil, mayonnaise	1 tsp.
Russian or Thousand Island Dressing	2 tsps.
French or Italian Dressing	1 Tbsp.

Olives	5 large
Avocado	⅛ of 1 medium
Dry Roasted Nuts:	
Almonds	6
Pecans	2
Peanuts	10 large
Walnuts	2
Sunflower or Sesame Seed	1 Tbsp.
Saturated Fats	
Butter	1 tsp.
Cream, light	2 Tbsp.
Cream, heavy	1 Tbsp.
Cream Cheese	1 Tbsp.
Sour Cream	2 Tbsp.
Bacon	1 slice
Salt Pork	¼ oz.

Diet and Shopping Tips

1. Take advantage of the "free" foods (no calories) allowed in the diabetic diet. Just a few raw vegetables, such as cucumbers and celery, taken at lunch and dinner can help satisfy the appetite while adding vitamins, minerals, enzymes and fiber to the diet.

2. Skip the oil on your salad and save on fat calories by using only vinegar or lemon juice. Try wine vinegar, cider vinegar and herb vinegars.

3. Fats can be reduced or eliminated by using non-stick cookware. These recipes will indicate where these utensils have been used and if there is a significant difference in fats.

4. Experiment with various herbs to help eliminate your salt craving.

5. Try drinking herbal teas. There is a large selection to choose from. Or add a pinch of cinnamon or nutmeg to your regular tea or coffee, a dash of vanilla extract instead of sweetener is also a zero calorie addition to tea.

6. "Dietetic" on a label does not mean "Diabetic." These foods are reduced in calories, but still may not be freely used. Also, there are many variations. The sodium content may be low, but the sugar content high, or the sugar content low while the fat content is high. Read the labels.

7. If you buy canned fruit, purchase only the unsweetened kind packed in its own juice. Fresh fruit is best as it has not gone through processing which can cause loss of vitamins and minerals.

8. Ideally, you should not buy packaged cookies, desserts or mixes. They compromise nutrition for empty calories. Home-made breads, nuts and fruit can satisfy your sweet tooth and wean you away from artificial sweeteners and processed products. But if you do buy processed or packaged items, always read the labels. In addition to brown sugar, sugar, corn syrup, corn sweetners, honey and molasses, the words dextrose, lactose, glucose, sorbitol and manitol mean sugar, These pack-aged foods and mixes can also contain unnecessary amounts of fats and sodium.

9. Buy sugar-free tomato sauce or make your own. In these recipes, you will find that a small amount goes a long way when used with other vegetables and herbs. If used indiscriminately, the calories can add up fast. One-quarter cup of tomato sauce equals 70 to 80 calories.

10. Beware of artificial sweeteners. Instead, try to get away from the craving for sugar. Not one study has shown that artifi-cial sweeteners help diabetics control their blood sugar or that they help dieters lose weight. In fact, some studies have shown that saccharin, for example, may actually stimulate the appe-tite and interfere with blood-sugar regulation. There is a cancer warning on products containing saccharin. In this world full of cancer causing substances, don't increase your chances.

11. If you buy fruit juice, pay attention to the name of the drink. The name "fruit juice" must by law contain 100 percent real fruit juice; a "juice drink" can have anywhere from 35 to 69 percent real juice; a "fruit drink" may contain only 10 to 34 percent juice; and a "fruit-flavored drink" which has less than 10 percent juice may often have no juice at all. Water, sugar, flavorings, and coloring take up the rest of the percentages.

12. Co-ops and bulk food buying clubs are a help to the vegetarian in that a wider variety of foods are available at lower prices. Most co-ops and natural food stores keep their produce in bins or crocks. You can scoop out as much as you need. Buy only enough to last a week or two. Unpreserved, unrefined grains, wheat germ and other cereals and nuts and seeds con-tain nutritious oils and should be refrigerated in a closed con-tainer to protect from rancidity and mold.

13. Remember: Eat on time.
Eat the proper amount for your diet.
Eat simple, nutritious foods.

Converting to a Vegetarian Exchange System

The vegetarian diet consists mainly of carbohydrates. Grains, vegetables, legumes and fruits are all in this category. Nuts and seeds are in the fats group, but are also important to the vegetarian diet. Certain combinations of these foods can provide as much or more protein than is found in the sources of concentrated or "complete" protein of meat or eggs.

Of the vegetable sources, legumes contain the greatest amount of protein. The highest amounts are found in mung beans and soybeans.

Grains contain the next highest amount of protein. Although they are not considered a main source of protein in the United States, they provide almost half of the protein in the world's diet. There are differences in the amount and quality that each kind supplies. Wheat, rye and oats have more protein by weight than corn, barley and millet. Oatmeal and buckwheat have the highest value of the grains and are comparable with beef.

Carrots, spinach, broccoli, and other "garden" vegetables contain some protein, but their main importance lies in being high-quality vitamin and mineral sources. The legume and grain combination is essential as the main protein source in the vegetarian diet, and vegetables serve as supplements. Fruits are not be considered protein sources at all, but are important to the vegetarian for vitamins, minerals and enzymes which activate the metabolic and assimilative processes.

None of these foods contain fat, which is an important consideration in today's society where obesity, heart problems and diabetes affect a large number of people. This brings us to nuts and seeds which are also an important source of protein in the vegetarian diet. Nuts and seeds do contain polyunsaturated fat which makes them high in calories. However, even with the high fat content, some nuts and seeds are so rich in protein that they are no more caloric per gram of usable protein than are the grains. The best are sesame and sunflower seeds, cashews and peanuts. Walnuts and pecans are higher in calories in proportion to their protein content, so should be used less frequently.

The lacto-ovo vegetarian diet, which allows use of dairy products and eggs ensures the vegetarian enough protein. Since vegetarians consume no saturated fats in their food, the fat content received from the moderate use of eggs, butter and low-fat or skim milk products would not be excessive.

Additional Vegetarian Exchanges*

Milk Exchanges

Soy Milk (add ½ bread exchange)	1 cup

Vegetable Exchanges

Alfalfa, mung or soybean sprouts, raw or cooked	1 cup

Fruit Exchanges

Carrot Juice	½ cup

Bread Exchanges

Brown Rice	⅓ cup (cooked)
Buckwheat Flour	3 Tbsp.
Bulghur	½ cup (cooked)
Cornmeal	2 Tbsp.
Millet	½ cup (cooked)
Oats	½ cup (cooked)
Pita Bread	½ of a 2 ½ oz. piece
Raw Bran	½ cup
Rice Flour	2 ½ Tbsp.
Rye Flour	2 ½ Tbsp.
Whole Wheat Flour	2 ½ Tbsp.

Meat Exchanges

Almond Butter	2 tsp.
Cashew Butter	2 tsp.
Peanuts (omit ½ bread and 2 fat exchanges)	4 Tbsp.
Soybeans	⅓ cup (cooked)
Soy Flour (omit 1 bread exchange)	¼ cup
Tahini	2 tsp. 2 tsp.
Tempeh	2 oz. (cooked)

Fat Exchanges

Tahini	1 tsp.

* Biermann, June & Touhey, Barbara, *The Diabetic's Total Health Book*, 1982, J.P. Tarcher, pp. 213-217

Combining Proteins

The proteins in our bodies are made up of combinations of 22 amino acids. Of these, nine cannot be synthesized by our bodies and must be obtained from our food. These must be consumed in balance with each other in order for protein formation to be complete. It's not necessary to eat foods that will provide the right amino acid complements at the same meal, but to insure that a balance is achieved it seems wise to get enough of each amino acid at mealtime. The vegetarian need only be concerned with understanding the relative balance of four amino acids, as these are essential to life functions, and if kept in balance, will contain the others in balance also. The four are: tryptophan, isoleucine, lysine, and the sulphur-containing amino acids.

In general, legumes with grains and nuts or seeds provide full complementation. Vegetables add to the protein quality as does the addition of small amounts of dairy products and eggs. It is a good idea to eat a wide variety of nuts, vegetables, grains, and legumes to obtain the benefit of the varying amounts of vitamins and minerals they contain.

Remember these basic combinations:

Grains with legumes	Legumes with dairy
Grains with seeds and nuts	products or eggs
Grains with dairy products	Seeds and nuts with
or eggs	legumes
Legumes with grains	Seeds and nuts with grains
Legumes with seeds and nuts	Seeds and nuts with dairy
	products or eggs

Once you understand the basic complement combinations, vegetarian meals can be made to fit into the exchange system. I do this by adding together all the calories of the ingredients in a recipe and then making the serving size according to the amount of calories allowed for the meal. Calories and nutritional value can be added to or decreased by changing the ingredients. For example:

Lentils + Rice—increase protein with sesame seed.

2 cups cooked brown rice = 464 calories

1 cup cooked lentils + 212 calories = 676 calories

2 servings, 338 calories each, 2½ meat, 2 bread exchanges each

add ¼ cup sesame seed = 203 calories

+ 676 calories = 879 calories

2 servings, 439 calories each, 3½ meat, 2 bread, 1 fat exchange each

Menu Planning

Since I take into consideration the fact that many vegetable sources from the starchy vegetable/bread group contain adequate amounts of protein, I place them in the meat exchange category as long as they are eaten in combination with another source containing complementary amino acids. In the same way, I consider nuts and seeds from the starchy vegetable/bread group to be a meat exchange also.

Another exchange of exchanges is to substitute foods in the starchy vegetable/bread group for those in the milk group. For example, in some snack and breakfast suggestions, I substitute 1 bread, 68 calories, in place of ½ cup lowfat milk, which is about the same amount of calories. Do not, however, substitute fruit or the non-starchy vegetables from group two for protein requirements. They are not good sources of protein and should be kept in their own exchange groups. Use only nuts or seeds from the fats group to count as protein too. Oils, butter and margarine contain no protein.

On the following pages is a sample 2-day ovo-lacto vegetarian menu with calories and exchanges given.

2 Day Menu for a 2000 Calorie Diet

Day 1

Breakfast
1 cup cooked oatmeal
1 cup low-fat milk
2 Tbsp. raisins
1 Tbsp. sunflower seeds

2 bread, ½ milk, 1 fruit,
  1 fat, 305 calories

Snack
1 banana

1 fruit, 100 calories

Lunch
2 slices whole wheat bread
2 oz. cheddar cheese
mustard
1 large apple
8 oz. plain yogurt
small green salad w/free
  dressing, p. 74

2 bread, 2 meat, 1 milk,
  590 calories

Day 1 (cont.)

Supper
Peanut Loaf, p. 104
small green salad w/free
dressing, p. 74
½ cup plain yogurt
1 cup cooked broccoli

*4 meat, 2 bread, 1½ fat, ½ milk,
2 vegetable, 635 calories*

Total Calories for Day 1 = 1,987

Snack
20 grapes
1 english muffin, p. 60
2 tsp. butter
1 oz. peanuts

*4 fat, 1 bread, 1 fruit,
339 calories*

Day 2

Breakfast
Bulghur Wheat, p. 55

*2½ bread, 1 fruit, 2 fat,
½ milk, 395 calories*

Snack
2 oranges
20 almonds

2 fruit, 2 fat

Lunch
Garbanzo-Noodle Salad
w/Yogurt, p. 71
20 grapes

*4 bread, 2 meat, 2 vegetable,
2½ fat, ¼-½ milk, 1 fruit,
461 calories*

Supper
Tofu-Vegie Pie, p. 88
1 cup steamed yellow squash
small green salad w/free
dressing, p. 74
1 piece whole wheat bread
1 tsp. butter

*3 bread, 3 meat, 2 vegetable,
2 fat, 550 calories*

Total Calories for Day 2 = 1,975

Snack
Popcorn w/peanuts and
raisins, p. 127
½ cup plain yogurt

*1 bread, 2 fruit, 2 fat, ½ milk,
369 calories*

Cooking Chart for Grains and Beans

1 cup dry	cups of water	cooking time	yield
Barley	3	1 hour	3½ cups
Black Beans	4	1½ hours	2 cups
Black-eyed Peas	3	1 hour	2 cups
Brown Rice	2	1 hour	3 cups
Buckwheat (kasha)	2	15 min.	2½ cups
Bulghur	2	15 min.	2½ cups
Garbanzo Beans	4	2 hours	2 cups
Great Northern Beans	3	2 hours	2 cups
Kidney Beans	3	1½ hours	2½ cups
Lentils and Split Peas	3	1 hour	2¼ cups
Lima Beans	2	1½ hours	1¼ cups
Millet	3	45 min.	3½ cups
Navy Pea Beans	3 cups	2½ hours	2 cups
Oatmeal	2 cups	5 min.	1½ cups
Pinto Beans	3 cups	2½ hours	2 cups
Soy Beans	3	2½ hours	2 cups
Soy Grits	4	15 min.	2 cups

Reprinted by permission from *The New Laurel's Kitchen,* by Laurel
Robertson, Carol Flinders and Brian Ruppenthal, copyright 1986, Ten Speed
Press, Berkeley, California

Weights and Measures

3 teaspoons = 1 Tablespoon = ½ fluid ounce
4 Tablespoons = ¼ cup = 2 fluid ounces
16 Tablespoons = 1 cup = 8 fluid ounces
2 Cups = 1 pint = 16 fluid ounces
2 Pints = 1 quart = 32 fluid ounces
4 Quarts = 1 gallon = 128 fluid ounces
2 Tablespoons = 1 ounce = ⅛ cup
4 Tablespoons = 2 ounces = ¼ cup
16 Tablespoons = 8 ounces = 1 cup
2 Cups = 16 ounces = 1 pound

Breakfast

Whole Wheat Blueberry Pancakes

Makes 12 pancakes

See photo, facing page.

Mix together in a medium bowl:
   2 cups whole wheat flour
   2 tsp. baking powder

Beat in:
   2 cups milk (low-fat)
   2 eggs
   1 Tbsp. oil

Stir in:
   1 cup blueberries

Lightly oil a frying pan and spoon batter on by tablespoons.

4 pancakes = 468 calories, 3 breads, 1 milk
Protein: 20 gm., Fat: 8 gm., Carbohydrates: 72 gm.

Buckwheat Pancakes

Makes 12 pancakes

Mix together in a medium bowl:
   1½ cups buckwheat flour
   1½ tsp. baking powder

Beat in:
   2 cups low-fat milk
   2 eggs
   2 Tbsp. oil

Lightly oil a frying pan. Spoon batter on by tablespoons.

4 pancakes = 363 calories, 3 breads, 1 milk, 1½ fat
Protein: 11 gm., Fat: 13 gm., Carbohydrates: 48 gm.

*In all the recipes in this book I will note the use of non-stick pans only if it will make a difference in the fat exchanges. It there is no note, the use of a non-stick pan will not change the amount of fats.

Whole Wheat Blueberry Pancakes, this page

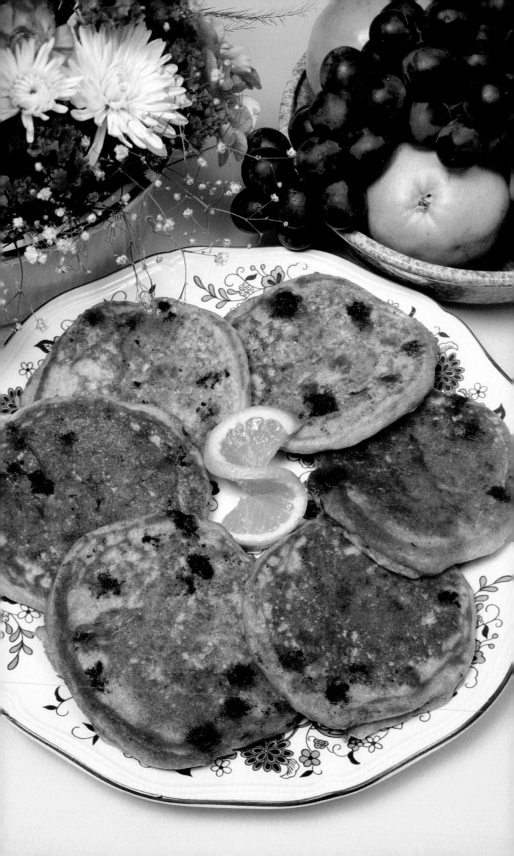

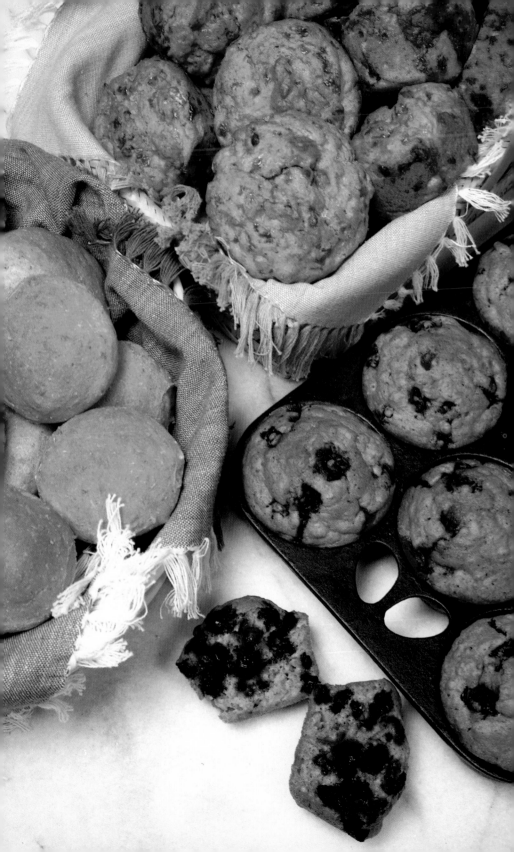

Raisin-Rice Cakes

Makes 9 cakes

A delicious pancake recipe without oil.

Mix together in a medium bowl:
1½ cups whole wheat pastry flour	1½ tsp. baking powder
1 cup cooked rice	1 tsp. cinnamon

Beat in:
    1½ cups milk
    1 egg

Stir in:
    ¼ cup raisins

Drop by tablespoons on lightly oiled frying pan. Cook on both sides.

1 serving of 3 = 382 calories each, 3 breads, 1 milk, 1 fruit
Protein: 16 gm., Fat: 2 gm., Carbohydrates: 71 gm.

Oatmeal Pancakes

Makes 9 pancakes

These pancakes are great for lunch sandwiches too. The oatmeal ones are especially good with peanut butter, and the buckwheat are good with cottage cheese.

Mix together in a medium bowl:
1½ cups oatmeal	2 tsp. baking powder
½ cup whole wheat flour	1 tsp. cinnamon

Beat in:
    1 cup low-fat milk
    1 egg
    1 Tbsp. oil
    ¼ cup raisins

Lightly oil a frying pan and spoon batter on by tablespoons turning when top bubbles.

3 pancakes = 484 calories, 3 breads, 1 fruit, 1 milk, 1 fat
Protein: 18 gm., Fat: 12 gm., Carbohydrates: 76 gm.

Herbed Wheat Rolls, p.59, Blueberry Oat Muffins, p.62, Strawberry Cottage-Cheese Muffins, p.63

Cornmeal-Soy Pancakes

Makes 12 pancakes

Mix together in a medium bowl:
    ¾ cup whole wheat pastry flour
    ¼ cup soy flour
    ½ cup cornmeal
    2 tsp. baking powder

Beat in:
    2 cups milk (low-fat)
    2 eggs
    2 Tbsp. oil

Lightly oil a frying pan and spoon batter on by tablespoons.

4 pancakes = 355 calories, 3 breads, 1 milk, 1 fat
Protein: 14 gm., Fat: 12 gm., Carbohydrates: 41 gm.

Breakfast Pudding

Makes 2 servings

Mix together and set aside in a small oven-proof bowl:
    ⅓ cup oatmeal
    1 cup low-fat milk
    1 egg
    1 banana, mashed
    1 tsp. vanilla

Set mixture aside to stand for 10 minutes to allow oatmeal to soak up flavor. Stir again and place in a small dish.

Preheat oven to 325°F.

Sprinkle with:
    cinnamon

Place dish in another oven-proof dish containing 1 inch of water. Bake for 15-20 minutes or until firm.

1 serving = 190 calories, ½ bread, 1 milk, 1 fruit; or ½ bread, ½ milk, ½ meat, 1 fruit
Protein: 8 gm., Fat: 3 gm., Carbohydrates: 30 gm.

BREAKFAST IN THE BLENDER

These drinks are a nutritious and satisfying way to start the day. If you add a couple of bread exchanges, breakfast can seem like a feast!

High Protein Vanilla Breakfast

This one is like an eggnog.

Blend in a blender until smooth and creamy:
   1 cup low-fat milk
   ¼ cup non-fat milk powder
   1 egg yolk
   1 tsp. vanilla
   ½ banana

1 serving = 297 calories, 1 milk, 2 meats, 1 fruit
Protein: 20 gm., Fat: 6 gm., Carbohydrates: 34 gm.

Creamy Peanut and Pineapple Shake

See photo, page 120.

This one is good with any juice or without the juice. Without the juice, you will be able to have a piece of fruit if your diet plan allows it at that meal.

Blend in a blender until smooth and creamy:
   1 cup low-fat milk
   ¼ cup low-fat milk powder
   1 Tbsp. peanut butter
   ½ tsp. vanilla
   ⅓ cup pineapple juice

1 serving = 311 calories, 1 milk, 2 meats, 1 fruit
Protein: 18 gm., Fat: 7 gm., Carbohydrates: 35 gm.

Blender Banana Breakfast

2 servings

Blend in a blender until smooth and creamy:
  1 cup low-fat milk
  ½ cup yogurt
  1 banana
  2 Tbsp. milk powder
  2 Tbsp. brewer's yeast

1 serving = 186 calories, 1 milk, 1 meat, 1 fruit
Protein: 16 gm., Fat: 3 gm., Carbohydrates: 27 gm.

CEREALS

Instead of corn flakes or cream of wheat, try adding other grains to your breakfast menu. Bulghur, millet, oats, buckwheat, brown rice, rye or wheat flakes, and barley can all be prepared for breakfast. Here are a few favorite combinations:

Brown Rice

Bring to a boil in a small saucepan:
  ⅔ cup water
  ⅓ cup brown rice

Simmer covered for 30 minutes. Remove from heat.

Add:
  2 chopped figs
  ¼ tsp. nutmeg

Serve in a bowl with:
  ¼ cup milk or yogurt (low-fat)

282 calories, 2 ½ breads, 1 fruit, ½ milk
Protein: 7 gm., Fat: 1 gm., Carbohydrates: 60 gm.

Bulghur Wheat

Bring to a boil in a small saucepan:
   ⅔ cup water
   ⅓ cup bulghur wheat

Simmer, covered, until liquid is absorbed.

Blend to a fine powder in a blender:
   2 Tbsp. cashews

Add and blend again:
   ½ tsp. vanilla
   ¼ cup milk or yogurt (low-fat)

Pour over bulghur and cook 5 more minutes.

Add:
   1 banana, sliced

387 calories, 2½ breads, 1 fruit, 2 fats, ½ milk
Protein: 10 gm., Fat: 3 gm., Carbohydrates: 71 gm.

Hot Oatmeal

Mix in a small pan:
   1 cup hot water
   ⅔ cup oatmeal

Cook gently for 5 to 6 minutes.

Add:
   1 Tbsp. raisins
   ½ tsp. cinnamon
   1 Tbsp. sunflower seeds

Serve with:
   ¼ cup milk or yogurt (low-fat)

352 calories, 2 breads, 1 fruit, 1 fat, ½ milk
Protein: 13 gm., Fat: 6 gm., Carbohydrates: 57 gm.

Baked Oatmeal

Makes 2 servings

Preheat oven to 350°F.

Mix in a small casserole dish in the order listed:
- 1½ cups oatmeal
- ¼ cup milk powder
- 1 banana, mashed
- 1½ cups hot water
- 1 Tbsp. oil

Bake for 20 minutes.

1 serving = 418 calories, 1 milk, 2 breads, 1 fat, 1 fruit
Protein: 14 gm., Fat: 13 gm., Carbohydrates: 66 gm.

Variation

Replace banana with:
- 2 Tbsp. raisins
- ¼ cup coconut

Sprinkle with:
- cinnamon

Bake for 20 minutes.

1 serving = 428 calories, 1 milk, 2 breads, 2 fats, 1 fruit
Protein: 14 gm., Fat: 16 gm., Carbohydrates: 61 gm.

Granola

Makes 7 cups

Oatmeal is the one grain which does not have to be cooked to be digested. By not cooking it, no vitamins are lost.

Mix together and store in airtight container in the refrigerator:

3 cups rolled oats	½ cup chopped dates
½ cup bran	1 cup chopped almonds
½ cup wheat germ	2 Tbsp. sesame seed
½ cup chopped raisins	

½ cup = 240 calories, 1 bread, 1 fruit, 2 fats
Protein: 8 gm., Fat: 4 gm., Carbohydrates: 35 gm.

Breads

Basic Whole Wheat Bread

Makes 2 loaves

A little bit of honey in a yeast bread makes the bread rise better. One tablespoon in a loaf of bread does not contribute significant calories. The bread can be made without it, but if you are new to working with whole wheat, you may find that you need help in getting it to rise the first few times. A little honey to help the yeast may be all you will need.

Stir together in a large bowl until the yeast is dissolved:
    1 Tbsp. honey
    1 Tbsp. yeast
    2½ cups warm water

Beat in:
    3 cups whole wheat flour

Mix in gradually:
    3 additional cups whole wheat flour

On a lightly floured surface, knead the dough until it is soft and springy. Form into 2 loaves and place in lightly oiled bread pans. Cover the pans with a clean towel. Let the bread rise until almost double in size. Bake at 350° F. for 45 minutes.
15 slices per loaf, each slice = 82 calories, 1 bread
Protein: 3 gm., Fat: 0 gm., Carbohydrates: 18 gm.

Half Whole Wheat Bread

Makes 2 loaves

Dissolve together:
    4 tsp. dry yeast
    1 cup lukewarm water
    1 tsp. honey

Set aside for 10 minutes.

Combine and set aside:
    4 cups whole wheat flour
    3 cups white unbleached flour

Mix together in a large bowl:
    ¼ cup honey
    ⅓ cup oil
    2 cups warm low-fat milk or soymilk
    the yeast mixture

Stir the flour mixture into the liquid ingredients in the large bowl to make a kneadable dough. Turn the dough onto a floured surface and knead for 10 minutes, adding more white flour if dough is too wet. Divide dough in half and place each half in an oiled bread pan. Cover pans with a towel and let the dough rise for 1½ hrs. Bake at 350° F. for 1 hour or until done.

One loaf = about 16 large slices, 123 calories per slice, 1½ bread exchanges or one low-fat milk exchange
Protein: 4 gm., Fat: 2 gm., Carbohydrates: 22 gm.

Herbed Wheat Rolls

Makes 10 rolls

See photo, page 50.

These little buns are great for accompanying a salad or a vegetable soup. Try melting cheese on them to bring out the herb flavor. (For each 1 oz. of cheese count 1 meat exchange)

Preheat oven to 350° F.

Heat in a small saucepan until warm:
    1 cup low-fat milk

Add:
    1 Tbsp. yeast
    2 tsp. butter

Beat in:
    1½ cups whole wheat flour
    ½ tsp. dill
    ½ tsp. oregano
    ½ tsp. thyme

Drop by tablespoons onto floured baking sheet, making 10 rolls. Bake about 15 minutes.

1 roll = 79 calories, 1 bread
Protein: 3 gm., Fat: 0 gm., Carbohydrates: 14 gm.

The Best English Muffins

Makes 12 4" muffins

This is our favorite bread. We like them best split and toasted or heated with cheese and sprouts in the oven.

Combine and set aside:
   2 Tbsp. yeast
   ½ cup flour

Heat in a small saucepan until warm:
   1¾ cups milk (low-fat)
   1 Tbsp. honey (optional)
   2 Tbsp. oil

Stir the yeast and flour into the milk mixture and mix until dissolved. Pour this into a large bowl.

Beat in:
   4 cups whole wheat or unbleached flour

Knead ten minutes on a lightly floured surface. Roll out the dough and cut into twelve 4-inch rounds. Place the rounds on a floured baking sheet. Let rise one hour. Bake at 350° F. for about 25 minutes.

1 muffin = 194 calories, 2 breads, 1 fat
Protein: 7 gm., Fat: 3 gm., Carbohydrates: 35 gm.

Cinnamon Raisin Muffins

Makes 12 muffins

Preheat oen to 400° F.

Mix together:
   2 cups whole wheat pastry flour
   2 tsp. baking powder
   1 tsp. cinnamon

Stir in:
   1 ½ oz. raisins
   ½ cup walnuts (optional)

Lightly beat:
   1 egg

Add to egg:
   1 ½ cups water
   ¼ cup oil
   1 Tbsp. honey

Stir liquids into dry ingredients, careful not to overmix. Spoon into oiled muffin tins. Bake for 15 minutes.

1 muffin = 164 calories, 1 bread, 1 fruit, 1 ½ fats
Protein: 4 gm., Fat: 8 gm., Carbohydrates: 19 gm.

Bran and Wheat Germ Muffins
Makes 12 muffins

The addition of a banana gives plenty of natural sweetness to these muffins without a lot of calories.

Preheat oven to 375° F.

Mix together in a medium mixing bowl:
   1 cup whole wheat pastry flour
   ½ cup bran
   ½ cup wheat germ
   1½ tsp. cinnamon
   2 tsp. baking powder

Stir in and avoid overmixing:
   ¼ cup powdered non-fat milk
   2 eggs
   2 Tbsp. oil
   1 banana, mashed

Fold in:
   ⅓ cup chopped walnuts

Spoon into lightly oiled muffin cups. Bake for 15-20 minutes.

1 muffin = 124 calories, 1 bread, 1½ fats
Protein: 5 gm., Fat: 5 gm., Carbohydrates: 14 gm.

Blueberry Oat Muffins

Makes 12 muffins

See photo, page 50.

Oatmeal gives these muffins a moist chewy texture that goes well with the blueberry flavor.

Mix together in a medium mixing bowl:
1 cup whole wheat pastry flour	**½ tsp. cinnamon**
1 cup rolled oats	**1 Tbsp. baking powder**

Stir in carefully and avoid overmixing:
- **1 cup milk (low-fat)**
- **1 egg**
- **1 Tbsp. honey**
- **2 Tbsp. oil**

Fold in:
- **1 cup blueberries**

Spoon into lightly oiled muffin cups. Bake for 15-20 minutes.

1 muffin = 117 calories, 1 bread, ½ fat, ½ fruit
Protein: 4 gm., Fat: 4 gm., Carbohydrates: 17 gm.

Egg-less Rye Muffins

Makes 12 muffins

Preheat oven 350° F.

Mix together in a medium mixing bowl:
- **2 cups light rye flour**
- **2 tsp. baking powder**
- **¼ cup powdered milk**

Stir in:
- **1 cup milk (low-fat)**
- **2 Tbsp. oil**

Spoon into lightly oiled muffin cups, making 12 muffins. Bake for 10-15 minutes.

1 muffin = 88 calories, 1 bread
Protein: 3 gm., Fat: 3 gm., Carbohydrates: 13 gm.

Strawberry-Cottage Cheese Muffins

Makes 12 muffins

See photo, page 50.

Preheat oven to 350° F.

Mix together in a large bowl:
> 2 cups unbleached white or whole wheat pastry flour
> 2 tsp. baking powder

Combine in a separate bowl:
> ¼ cup white sugar or honey
> 1 cup low-fat cottage cheese
> ½ cup cold water
>
> 1 tsp. vanilla
> 1 egg
> ¼ cup oil

Stir the wet ingredients into the dry ingredients until moistened. Stir in:
> 1 cup chopped fresh strawberries

Pour into lightly oiled muffin pans and bake for about 15 minutes.

1 muffin = 152 calories, 1 bread, 1 fruit, ½ fat exchange)
Protein: 5 gm., Fat: 5 gm., Carbohydrates: 20 gm.

Cornmeal Rice Buns

Makes 9 buns

Preheat oven to 375° F.

Combine in a medium bowl, stirring until smooth:
> 1 cup boiling water
> 1¼ cups cornmeal
> 2 Tbsp. soy flour

Mix in:
> 1 cup cooked rice
> 2 Tbsp. oil

Form 9 patties. Bake on floured baking sheet 25-30 minutes.

1 bun = 115 calories, 1 bread, 1 fat
Protein: 2 gm., Fat: 4 gm., Carbohydrates: 18 gm.

Buttermilk French Toast

Makes 6 slices

Beat together:
   2 eggs
   ½ cup buttermilk
   ¼ cup water

Arrange in a shallow baking dish:
   6 slices whole wheat bread

Pour egg and buttermilk mixture over bread slices. Cover and allow to soak for at least ½ hour.

When ready to cook, brown 3 slices at a time in:
   1 tsp. butter.
For non-stick pan, use no butter and eliminate fat exchange.

1 serving of 3 slices = 287 calories, 3 breads, 1 meat, 1 fat; or 2 breads, ½ milk, 1 meat, 1 fat
Protein: 16 gm., Fat: 5 gm., Carbohydrates: 37 gm.

Apple-Oat Drop Cookies

Makes 20 cookies

See photo, page 68.

Mash together with a fork:
   1½ cups oatmeal
   1 Tbsp. whole wheat flour
   2 medium apples, grated
   1 Tbsp. oil
   ½ tsp. vanilla
   ¼ cup water

Mix in:
   ½ cup raisins
   ¼ cup finely chopped walnuts

Let the mixture soak together in the bowl for 15 minutes. Preheat oven to 350° F. Drop by tablespoons onto an ungreased baking sheet. Bake for 10-12 minutes.

1 cookie = 63 calories, ½ bread, ½ fruit
Protein: 2 gm., Fat: 21 gm., Carbohydrates: 10 gm.

Sesame-Cornmeal Biscuits

Makes 12 biscuits

See photo on the cover.

Preheat oven to 350° F.

Mix together throughly in a medium mixing bowl:
    1 cup whole wheat pastry flour   2 tsp. baking powder
    ⅔ cup cornmeal   1 Tbsp. sesame seeds
    ⅓ cup wheat germ

Add and beat well:
    1 Tbsp. oil
    1 cup low-fat milk

Drop onto floured cookie sheet by tablespoons, making 12 biscuits.
Bake 20-25 minutes.

1 biscuit = 92 calories, 1 bread, ½ fat
Protein: 4 gm., Fat: 2 gm., Carbohydrates: 15 gm.

Banana-Raisin Bran Biscuits

Makes 12 biscuits

Preheat oven to 350° F.

Mix together in a medium mixing bowl:
    1½ cups whole wheat pastry flour
    ½ cup bran
    2 tsp. baking powder

Stir in:
    ½ cup milk (low-fat)
    1 egg
    1 tsp. vanilla
    1 banana, mashed

Add:
    ½ cup raisins
    ½ cup chopped walnuts

Drop onto ungreased cookie sheet, making 12 biscuits. Bake for 15
minutes.

1 biscuit = 126 calories, 1 bread, 1 fruit
Protein: 5 gm., Fat: 3 gm., Carbohydrates: 20 gm.

Energy Biscuits

Makes 30 biscuits

Preheat oven to 325° F.

Mix together in a large mixing bowl:

1 cup cornmeal	½ cup soy flour
½ cup whole wheat flour	½ cup wheat germ
½ cup rye flour	½ cup bran

Add and beat well:
   ¼ cup nonfat milk powder
   1 cup water
   1 egg

Lightly oil a 9" x 13" pan and press dough in evenly. Bake for about 25 minutes. Allow bread to cool then cut into 30 pieces.

2 pieces = 95 calories, 1 bread
Protein: 5 gm., Fat: 1 gm., Carbohydrates: 16 gm.

Nutritional Yeast Gravy or Sauce

This is a tasty vegetarian gravy for biscuits and many other dishes.

Combine in a sauce pan:
   ⅓ cup yeast
   ⅓ cup flour
   2 cups water

Cook over low heat until bubbling. Remove from heat.

Add:
   1 Tbsp. butter
   1 tsp. prepared mustard

For a darker sauce, mix the flour and yeast in a saucepan and brown first.

2 Tbsp. = 17 calories, ½ bread or ½ meat
Protein: 0 gm., Fat: 0 gm., Carbohydrates: 2 gm.

Garbanzo-Vegetable Soup, p.77, Apple-Oat Drop Cookies, p. 64

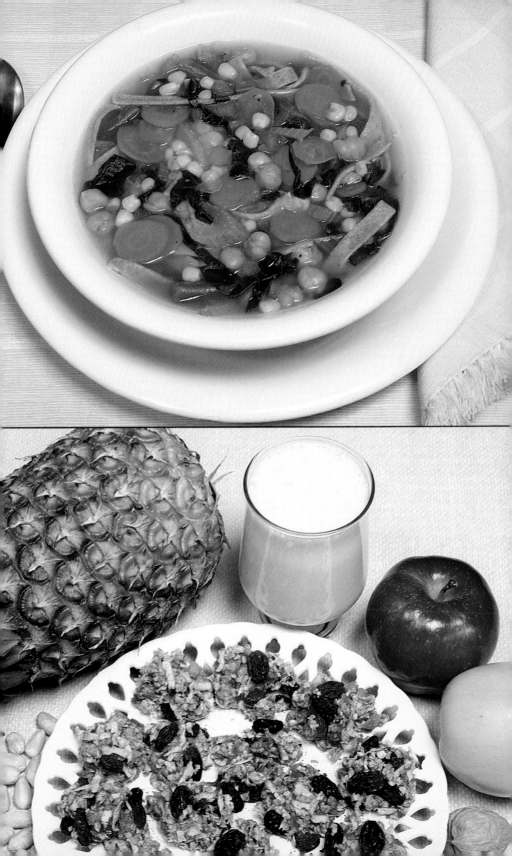

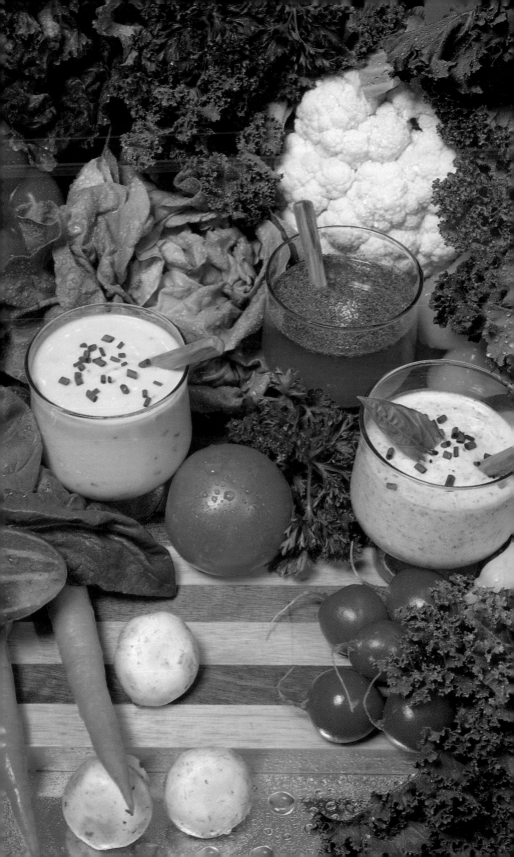

Salads and Salad Dressings

Yogurt Mock Russian, Lemon-Tomato Juice Dressing, Herbed Yogurt Thoroughly, p. 73, Basic Free Dressing, p. 74

SALADS

Basic Free Green Salad

Enjoy up to 2 cups free!

See photo on back cover.

2 cups shredded romaine lettuce
2 cups shredded iceberg lettuce
1 cup shredded spinach or swiss chard
12 sliced or whole radishes

1 cup curly endive
1 sliced cucumber
2 stalks celery, diced,
   with tops

Other ingredients to form your own combinations:
boston or bibb lettuce
shredded red or green cabbage
kale or comfrey
chicory or sorrell
lambsquarters leaves
parsley or watercress
turnip, collard, mustard,
   dandelion, or beet greens
green or wax beans
onions, tomatoes, sprouts

sliced fresh mushrooms
sliced fresh red or green
  peppers
flowerettes of broccoli
  or cauliflower
slices of zucchini or yellow
squash
brussels sprouts, halved
  or quartered
scallions or chives

Vegetarian "Chef's Salad"

Any of the dressings are good with this salad, but our favorite is the tahini.

Mix in a large individual salad bowl:
    2 cups basic free salad

Add:
    2 Tbsp. diced cheddar cheese
    2 Tbsp. diced Swiss cheese
    ¼ cup cold garbanzo beans
    2 Tbsp. peanuts

Top with:
    1 slice toasted whole wheat bread, cut into crouton-sized
cubes

3 meat exchanges, 2 fat exchanges and 1 bread exchange
Protein: 20 gm., Fat: 8 gm., Carbohydrates: 31 gm.

Tofu Salad I

See photo on the cover.

Mix together:

7 oz. tofu, diced	½ cup chopped tomato
¼ cup cottage cheese	¼ cup chopped peppers and onions

Place on a bed of lettuce, garnish with cucumber slices and alfalfa sprouts.

1 serving = 228 calories, 4 meats, 1 vegetable
Protein: 23 gm., Fat: 10 gm., Carbohydrates: 12 gm.

Tofu Salad II

Mix together:
   6 oz. tofu, diced
   1 Tbsp. tahini

Stir in:

½ cup chopped tomato	¼ cup finely diced carrots
¼ cup chopped peppers and onions	¼ cup sprouts

Place on a bed of lettuce.

Protein: 20 gm., Fat: 28 gm., Carbohydrates: 15 gm.

Garbanzo-Noodle Salad With Yogurt

Makes 2 servings

Mix together:

1 cup cooked garbanzos	1 cup steamed broccoli, chopped
2 cups cooked whole wheat noodles	1 cup steamed carrots, chopped
	1 Tbsp. sesame tahini
2 Tbsp. chopped onions	1 Tbsp. lemon juice

Top with:
   ½-1 cup plain yogurt

1 serving = 447 calories, 2 meats, 2 breads, 2 vegetables, 1 fat, + ¼ -½ milk exchanges
Protein: 24 gm., Fat: 12 gm., Carbohydrates: 69 gm.

Tofu Potato Salad

Makes 1 serving

This tofu salad makes a great hot weather dish.

Steam and dice:
   1 large potato (1 cup)

Mix together in a medium bowl with the diced potato:

6 oz. tofu, diced	¼ tsp. rosemary
¼ cup low-fat cottage cheese	1 tsp. tarragon
½ cup diced tomato	¼ tsp. ground bay leaves
2 Tbsp. chopped onion	¼ tsp. basil
2 Tbsp. chopped pepper	1 Tbsp. sunflower seeds
½ cup alfalfa sprouts	1 oz. unsalted peanuts
½ tsp. oregano	1 tsp. mayonnaise

Serve on a bed of lettuce.

1 serving = 539 calories, 4 meats, 2 breads, 1½ fats, 1 vegetable
Protein: 35 gm., Fat: 17 gm., Carbohydrates: 36 gm.

Sprouts

These beans and seeds can be sprouted:

wheat or rye berries	mung beans
sunflower seeds	soybeans
sesame seeds	lentils
alfalfa seeds	watercress seeds
radish seeds	garbanzo beans

Rinse beans or seeds and put about 2 Tbsp. in a quart jar with water and let soak overnight or at least six hours. Cover top with cheese cloth or sprouting jar covers (which can be found in many department stores). After soaking time is up, drain the water through the covers or cloth. Rinse two or three times a day to keep sprouts moist. They will begin to sprout in one or two days and will be fully sprouted in four to five days. Keep them in the refrigerator after they are fully sprouted and use promptly.

SALAD DRESSINGS

Yogurt Mock Russian

See photo, page 67.

Mix together thoroughly:

2 Tbsp. sugar-free ketchup
1 cup yogurt (low-fat)
¼ cup water
1 clove garlic, minced

2 Tbsp. chopped dill pickle
2 Tbsp. chopped chives
½ tsp. mustard powder
½ tsp. tamari

1-2 Tbsp. = Free
1 Tbsp. = Calories: 8, Carbohydrates: 1 gm.

Lemon-Tomato Juice Dressing

See photo on back cover.

Mix together thoroughly:

1 cup tomato juice
2 Tbsp. lemon juice
1 tsp. basil

1 tsp. bay
2 Tbsp. chopped onion
1 Tbsp. chopped parsley

1-2 Tbsp. = Free
1 Tbsp. = Calories: 4, Carbohydrates: 1 gm.

Herbed Yogurt Thoroughly

See photo, page 67.

Mix together thoroughly:

1 cup yogurt (low-fat)
4 Tbsp. chives
1 tsp. tarragon
1 tsp. dill

½ tsp. bay
½ tsp. basil
½ tsp. marjoram
1 Tbsp. lemon juice

1-2 Tbsp. = Free
1 Tbsp. = Calories: 8, Carbohydrates: 1 gm.

Herbed Olive Oil Dressing

Mix together thoroughly:

⅓ cup olive oil
3 Tbsp. wine vinegar
2 Tbsp. chopped parsley

¼ tsp. kelp powder
¼ tsp. pepper
Enough water to make 1 cup

1 Tbsp. = 1 fat
Calories: 40, Fat: 1 gm.

Tahini Dressing

Mix together thoroughly:

1 cup sesame tahini
3 Tbsp. lemon juice
⅔ cup water

1 Tbsp. minced onion
1 clove garlic, minced

1 Tbsp. = 1 fat
Calories: 56, Protein: 2 gm., Fat: 10 gm., Carbohydrates: 1 gm.

Basic Free Dressing

See photo, page 67.

Mix together thoroughly:

½ cup cider or wine vinegar
½ cup water
½ tsp. dry mustard

½ tsp. pepper
1 tsp. celery seed
1 tsp. dill seed

Free
1 Tbsp. = Calories: 1

Soups and Sandwiches

SOUPS

All kinds of combinations of beans, grains, and vegetables can be put together for soup. Here are six of our favorites.

Tofu Vegetable Soup

One serving

Cook for 15 minutes:
  2 Tbsp. uncooked brown rice
  2 cups water

Add and simmer 10-15 minutes longer:
  ¾ cup carrots, sliced   ½ cup onions, chopped
  1 small potato, diced   Tarragon, bay, basil, celery
  ¼ cup fresh or frozen peas   seed to taste
  ½ cup celery, sliced

Stir in:
  8 oz. firm tofu, cut into bite-size pieces

1 serving = 407 calories, 4 meats, 2 breads, 2 vegetables
Protein: 25 gm., Fat: 10 gm., Carbohydrates: 57 gm.

Pea Soup

Four 1½ cup servings

Cook for 1 hour:
  ½ cup dried split peas
  ¼ cup barley, uncooked
  6 cups of water, coveed

Add, cover and cook another 30 minutes:
  1 cup diced potato   1 cup carrots, diced
  1 cup chopped onions   bay, basil, tarragon,
  1 cup shredded cabbage   pepper to taste
  1 stalk celery, diced

1 serving = 272 calories, 2 meats, 2 breads, 2 vegetables
Protein: 10 gm., Fat: 0 gm., Carbohydrates: 58 gm.

Garbanzo-Vegetable Soup

Four servings

See photo, page 68.

Have ready:
   ½ cup cooked garbanzo beans

Bring to a boil in a 2 quart saucepan and simmer, covered, for 10 minutes:

½ cup fresh or frozen corn	1 cup shredded spinach
½ cup fresh or frozen	or cabbage
green beans	2 cups water
½ cup carrots, diced	parsley, oregano, basil,
½ cup celery, diced	bay leaves to taste
¼ cup chopped onions	

Add:

1 tsp. tomato sauce	¼ cup uncooked whole wheat
the cooked garbanzo beans	or enriched noodles

Simmer 5 more minutes, until noodles are cooked.

1 serving = 368 calories, 3 meats, 2 breads, 2 vegetables
Protein: 22 gm., Fat: 0 gm., Carbohydrates: 70 gm.

Easy Lentil Stew

Six servings

Cook for about 1 hour:

1 cup lentils, uncooked	thyme, oregano, pepper to taste
1 cup brown rice, uncooked	6 cups water

Add more water if needed.

Add and cook another 15 minutes:

2 cups diced carrots	1 medium tomato, chopped
1 cup chopped onion	1 cup shredded spinach
2 stalks celery with tops,	(optional)
diced	

1 serving = 204 calories, 2 meats, 2 breads, 2 vegetables
Protein: 14 gm., Fat: 0 gm., Carbohydrates: 62 gm.

Creamy Garbanzo Soup

Four servings

Cook until the beans are soft (about 2 hours):
    1½ cups uncooked garbanzo beans   ½ cup chopped celery
    2 cups chopped onion   ½ cup diced carrots

Puree in a blender then return to the pot.

Stir in:
    2 cups low-fat milk
    ¼ cup milk powder

Steam and add to the soup:
    1 ½ cup diced carrots

Season to taste with:
    pepper, parsley and kelp

1 serving = 401 calories, 4 meats, 1 bread
Protein: 23 gm., Fat: 2 gm., Carbohydrates: 67 gm.

Tofu-Tomato Soup

Two servings

Cook for 30-40 minutes:
    ½ cup uncooked brown rice
    1½ cups water

In a separate saucepan simmer for 10 minutes:
    4 medium tomatoes, chopped   ½ tsp. pepper
    ½ cup chopped onion   ½ tsp. kelp
    ½ tsp. basil   1 Tbsp. butter

Puree vegetables in blender and set aside.

In a large pot, stir together:
    2 Tbsp. whole wheat flour
    ¼ cup low-fat milk powder
    2 cups low-fat milk

Add and heat:
   8 oz. tofu, diced
   the cooked rice
   the tomato puree

Simmer, stirring every few minutes.

Stir in:
   1 Tbsp. parsley or chives

1 serving = 482 calories, 2 meats, 2 breads, 1 milk, 1½ fats, 2 vegetables
Protein: 27 gm., Fat: 12 gm., Carbohydrates: 61 gm.

SANDWICHES

Four Great Cottage Cheese Sandwiches

Makes 2 sandwiches each

These are good on basic whole wheat bread, but try having them in Syrian flat breads, or as open-face sandwiches heated up in the oven. On hot days these combinations make a cool lunch when served on a bed of lettuce with crackers or muffins on the side.

1. ½ cup cottage cheese (low-fat)
   2 Tbsp. peanut butter
   1 sandwich = 141 calories, 2 meats, 2 fats; or 3 meats
   Protein: 11 gm., Fat: 4 gm., Carbohydrates: 6 gm.

2. ¼ cup cottage cheese (low-fat)
   1 hard boiled egg
   ¼ cup alfalfa sprouts
   1 tsp. mayonnaise (optional)
   1 chopped dill pickle
   70 calories, 2 meats, 1 fat
   Protein: 8 gm., Fat: 2 gm., Carbohydrates: 2 gm.

3. ¼ cup cottage cheese (low-fat)
   2 tsp. chives
   2 tbsp grated cheddar cheese
   ¼ finely diced celery
   56 calories, 2 meats
   Protein: 6 gm., Fat: 2 gm., Carbohydrates: 1 gm.

4. ¼ cup cottage cheese (low-fat)
   2 Tbsp. raisins
   2 Tbsp. cashews, chopped
   ½ tsp. cinnamon
   1 sandwich = 104 calories, 2 meats, 2 fats, 2 fruits
   Protein: 6 gm., Fat: 2 gm., Carbohydrates: 11 gm.

Four Great Bean-based Sandwiches

These also make good sandwiches for traveling. The tempeh-tomato-cheese sandwich is good when heated in the oven.

1. ¼ cup cooked pinto beans, mashed
    2 tsp. tomato sauce
    1 tsp. chopped onion
    2 Tbsp. grated cheddar cheese
    shredded lettuce
    115 calories, 2 meats, 1 fruit
    Protein: 7 gm., Fat: 3 gm.,
    Carbohydrates: 11 gm.

2. ¼ cup cooked garbanzo beans, mashed
    2 tsp. sesame tahini
    1 tsp. chopped onion
    pinch garlic powder
    1 tsp. lemon juice
    164 calories, 1½ meats, 1 fat
    Protein: 7 gm., Fat: 14 gm.,
    Carbohydrates: 17 gm.

3. 6 oz. tofu, diced
    2 tsp. sesame tahini
    ¼ cup alfalfa sprouts
    210 calories, 1 meats, 1 fat
    Protein: 17 gm., Fat: 21 gm.,
    Carbohydrates: 7 gm.

4. 2 oz. sliced tempeh, steamed
    1 oz. swiss cheese slice
    slice of tomato
    224 calories, 1½ meats, 1 fat
    Protein: 19 gm., Fat: 10 gm.,
    Carbohydrates: 4 gm.

Eight Great Peanut Butter Sandwiches

Makes 2 sandwiches each unless otherwise noted.

These spreads are best cold. They make good fillings for taking to work or school.

1. 2 Tbsp. peanut butter
    2 tsp. sesame tahini
    1 Tbsp. sunflower seeds
    2 chopped figs
    1 sandwich = 184 calories
    2 meats, 3 fats, 1 fruit
    Protein: 7 gm., Fat: 11 gm.,
    Carbohydrates: 15 gm.

2. 2 Tbsp. peanut butter
    ¼ cup chopped celery
    2 Tbsp. yogurt
    2 Tbsp. peanuts, chopped
    1 sandwich = 150 calories
    2 meats, 2 fats
    Protein: 7 gm., Fat: 6 gm.,
    Carbohydrates: 7 gm.

3. 2 Tbsp. peanut butter
    2 Tbsp. grated cheddar
    cheese
    1 sandwich = 105 calories
    2 meats, 2 fats; or 3 meats
    Protein: 6 gm., Fat: 5 gm.,
    Carbohydrates: 4 gm.

4. ¼ cup tahini
    ¼ cup peanut butter
    ¼ cup raisins
    2 Tbsp. milk powder
    2 Tbsp. sunflower seeds
    1 sandwich = 513 calories
    2 meats, 1 fruit
    Protein: 19 gm., Fat: 47 gm.,
    Carbohydrates: 29 gm.

5. 2 Tbsp. peanut butter
    ½ banana, mashed
    2 Tbsp. non-fat milk powder
    ½ tsp. vanilla
    1 sandwich = 128 calories
    2½ meats, 1 fruit
    Protein: 6 gm., Fat: 4 gm.,
    Carbohydrates: 12 gm.

6. 2 Tbsp. peanut butter
    ¼ cup alfalfa sprouts
    1 Tbsp. sesame seeds
    8 or 10 slices cucumber
    1 tsp. mayonnaise
    1 sandwich = 132 calories
    2 meats, 2 fats
    Protein: 6 gm., Fat: 5 gm.,
    Carbohydrates: 5 gm.

7. 2 Tbsp. peanut butter
    2 Tbsp. raisins
    ¼ apple, chopped
    1 sandwich = 124 calories
    2 meats, 2 fruits
    Protein: 4 gm., Fat: 4 gm.,
    Carbohydrates: 13 gm.

8. 8 oz. tofu, mashed
    ¼ cup peanut butter
    1 banana, mashed
    1 tsp. lemon juice
    1 sandwich = 309 calories
    1 meat, ¼ fruit
    Protein: 18 gm., Fat: 12 gm.,
    Carbohydrates: 23 gm.

Tofu Pita Pizzas

See photo on back cover and page 85.

Preheat oven to 325° F.

Separate into two halves and place on a baking sheet:
    1 2-oz. pita bread

Mix together:
    6 oz. firm tofu, diced
    ½ cup chopped mushrooms
    4 thin slices onions
    4 thin slices green pepper
    2 Tbsp. tomato sauce

Top with:
    3 Tbsp. parmesan cheese

Bake for 10-15 minutes.

2 halves = 343 calories, 4 meats, 2 breads, 1 vegetable, ½ milk
Protein: 26 gm., Fat: 10 gm., Carbohydrates: 33 gm.

Crunchy Peanut Garbanzo Pitas

Mix together:
    ½ cup cooked garbanzo beans   2 Tbsp. crumbled feta cheese
    ½ cup diced celery   2 tsp. tahini
    ¼ cup alfalfa sprouts   1 tsp. tamari (optional)
    2 Tbsp. peanuts

Slice open:
    1 2-oz. pita bread

Fill pita bread with crunchy peanut mix. Serve hot or cold.

1 sandwich = 484 calories, 2 meats, 1 bread, 1 vegetables, ¼ milk
Protein: 23 gm., Fat: 16 gm., Carbohydrates: 51 gm.

Ratatouille Pitas

Preheat oven to 325° F.

Simmer in a medium saucepan until tender:
    1 Tbsp. chopped onion   ½ cup diced zucchini or eggplant
    ½ cup diced tomato   2 Tbsp. water
    ¼ cup alfalfa sprouts

Remove from heat.

Mix in:
    ¼ swiss or cheddar cheese, grated
    1 Tbsp. parmesan cheese, grated

Slice open:
    1 2-oz. pita bread

Fill the pita bread with ratatouille mix. Wrap in foil and heat in oven until thoroughly warm—about 5 minutes.

1 sandwich = 308 calories, 2½ meats, 2 breads, 2 vegetables
Protein: 19 gm., Fat: 6 gm., Carbohydrates: 32 gm.

Main Dishes

TOFU, TEMPEH, & SOYBEANS

Cashew-Carrot Parmesan

Three servings

Simmer:
> ½ cup uncooked millet
> 1 ½ cup water
> 1 tsp. oregano

In a separate medium saucepan simmer for 5 minutes:
> ½ cup diced carrots
> ½ cup chopped onions
> ½ cup water
> ½ tsp. oregano
> 1 tsp. broth powder

Drain cooking water from the vegetables into the millet and keep on low heat until the water is absorbed.

Preheat oven to 350° F.

Mix into vegetables:
> ½ cup cashews, broken

Add:
> the cooked millet
> 9 oz. tofu, sliced ½ thick

Place in an ungreased 1 qt. casserole dish.

Sprinkle with:
> 3 Tbsp. parmesan cheese

Bake for 10-15 minutes.

1 serving = 293 calories, 3 meats, 1 ½ breads, 1 veg., 1 fat
Protein: 15 gm., Fat: 7 gm., Carbohydrates: 26 gm.

Tofu Pita Pizzas, page 81

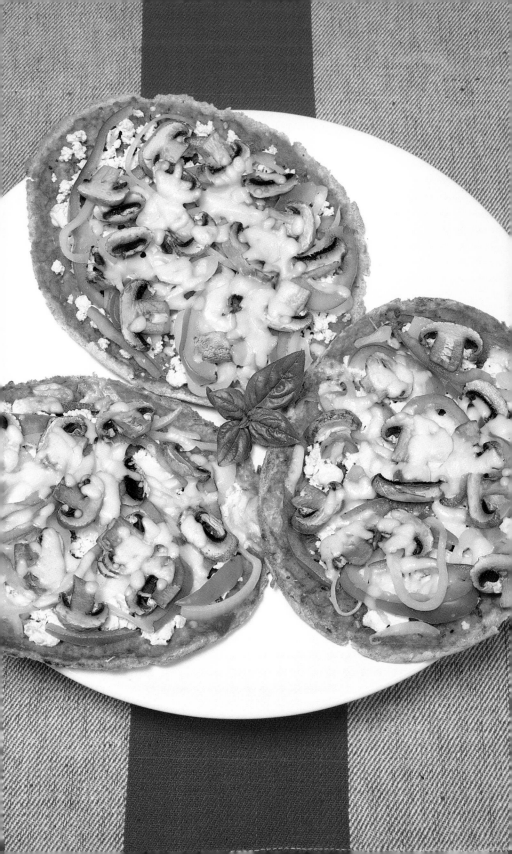

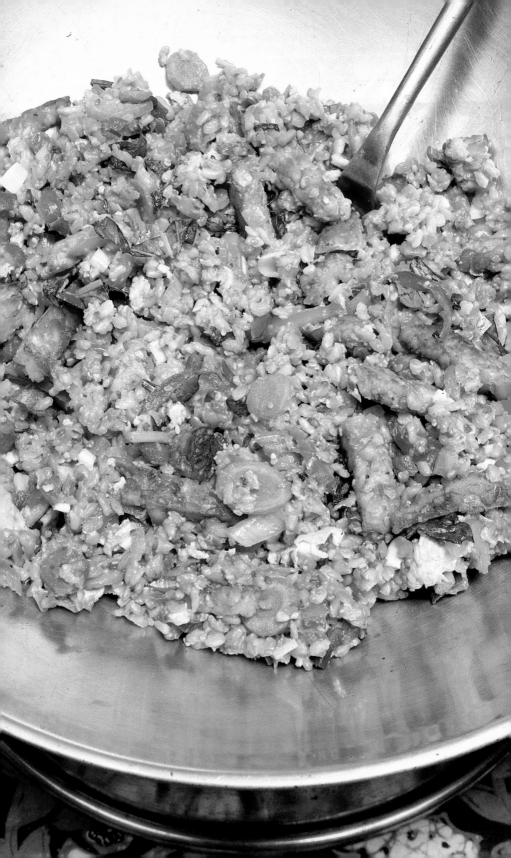

Far East Fried Rice

Two servings

See photo facing page.

Cut into julienne strips:
    8 oz. tofu or 8 oz. tempeh (steammed for 10 minutes and cooled)

Simmer for 45 minutes until liquid is absorbed:
    ½ cup brown rice
    1 ½ cups water

Heat in wok or skillet:
    1 Tbsp. oil

Add and brown lightly:
    2 Tbsp. sesame seeds

Add and brown:
    the tofu or tempeh

Stir in:
    ¼ cup onions, sliced
    ½ cup celery, sliced
    4 spinach leaves, shredded

Saute a few minutes, then add:
    the cooked rice

For extra protein you can make well in center of pan and drop in:
    1 egg (optional)

Cook a little, then mix egg with rice and vegetables.

Mix all ingredients together and add:
    4 tsp. tamari

Sprinkle on top to serve:
    ¼ cup green onions, chopped

1 serving = 347 calories, 4 meats, 2 breads, 2 fats
Protein: 14 gm., Fat: 13 gm., Carbohydrates: 36 gm.

Far East Fried Rice, page this page

Savory Tofu Casserole

Four servings

For non-stick pan, eliminate oil, eliminate ½ fat.

Preheat oven to 350° F.

Simmer together for 5 minutes:
     ½ cup chopped onion
     1 ½ cups chopped mushrooms
     ½ tsp. each tarragon, oregano & sage
     2 cups water

Mix in:
     2 cups oatmeal
     1 Tbsp. nutritional yeast
     1 lb. tofu, diced
     2 eggs

Grease an 8″ x 8″ casserole dish with:
     1 Tbsp. oil

Place mixture in dish and bake, covered, for 25 minutes.

Remove cover and top with:
     4 oz. cheese
     3 Tbsp. sunflower seeds

Return to oven and bake uncovered for 5 minutes more.

1 serving = 598 calories, 4 meats, 2 breads, ½ fat
Protein: 32 gm., Fat: 21 gm., Carbohydrates: 56 gm.

Tofu-Vegie Pie

Four servings

Simmer until tender (about 10 minutes):
     1 cup mixture chopped tomatoes, onions & peppers
     ¼ cup water

Preheat oven to 350° F.

Drain and pour excess water over:
  1 cup oatmeal

Mix oatmeal with:
  1 Tbsp. oil

Press into an 8″ pie plate. Bake for 10 minutes.

Combine:
  4 oz. cheese, grated
  the hot vegetables

Add and beat well:
  2 eggs, lightly beaten
  12 oz. tofu, diced

Fill crust with mixture.

Top with:
  2 Tbsp. sunflower seeds

Return to the oven for 15 minutes at 350° F. or until firm.

1 serving = 418 calories, 3½ meats, 2 breads, 1 fat
Protein: 23 gm., Fat: 17 gm., Carbohydrates: 29 gm.

Oriental Tofu

One serving

Simmer for 5 minutes:
  1 cup mushrooms, sliced or halved
  ½ cup sliced onions
  ½ cup water

Add and cook about 35 minutes more until rice is tender:
  ⅓ cup uncooked brown rice
  ⅓ cup water
  1 tsp. tamari

Add and cook another 5 minutes:
  6 oz. firm tofu, diced

1 serving = 357 calories, 3 meats, 2 breads, 2 vegetables
Protein: 20 gm., Fat: 8 gm., Carbohydrates: 53 gm.

Tofu-Mushroom Pot Pies

Four servings

Crust

Mix together with a fork:
- 1¼ cup whole wheat pastry flour
- ¼ cup wheat germ
- 3 Tbsp. oil
- 2-3 Tbsp. water

Break into 4 pieces and roll out each piece.

Filling

Simmer for 10 minutes:
- 2 cups chopped mushrooms
- 1 cup chopped celery with leaves
- 1 Tbsp. salt-free bouillon powder
- ½ cup water
- ½ cup chopped onion

Preheat oven to 350° F.

Stir in:
- 12 oz. tofu, diced

Divide filling into 4 oven proof dishes.

Slice into four pieces:
- 3 oz. cheese

Top each pie with cheese slice.

Bake for 30 minutes.

1 serving = 417 calories, 4 meats, 2 breads, 1 fat
Protein: 21 gm., Fat: 19 gm., Carbohydrates: 37 gm.

Tofu Quiche

This is similar to a quiche, and as with other recipes, experiment with different herbs and vegetables.

Simmer until liquid is absorbed:

⅔ cup brown rice	¼ tsp. bay leaves, ground
1 ½ cup water	¼ tsp. basil
¼ tsp. pepper	¼ tsp. thyme

Preheat oven to 350° F.

Toast for 5-10 minutes in the oven and set aside:
    ¼ cup sesame seeds

Add to cooked rice:
    1 tsp. butter

Press rice into a 9" pie plate and bake for 15 minutes.

Process or mash together:

9 oz. tofu, mashed	1 cup cashews, ground
½ cup green onions, chopped	1 egg (optional)

If tofu is very firm, process in 2 Tbsp. water to make spreading into shell easier)

Fill pie shell and top with sesame seeds. Bake at 350° F. for 20 minutes.

1 serving = 403 calories, 3 meats, 2 breads, 1 fat
Protein: 15 gm., Fat: 8 gm., Carbohydrates: 35 gm.

Tofu Pizza

Four servings

Crust

Preheat oven to 350° F.

Dissolve together:
   ½ cup warm water
   1 Tbsp. yeast

Mix in:
   1 cup whole wheat flour
   ⅓ cup oatmeal

Beat the mixture well. Roll out dough and place in a lightly oiled and floured pie plate and bake for 15 minutes.

Topping

Mix together:
   9 oz. diced tofu
   ⅓ cup tomato sauce
   5 Tbsp. parmesan cheese

When crust is ready, pour on tofu mixture and top with:
   4 oz. mozzarella, grated

You can also add a few sliced green peppers, onions or mushrooms along with the cheese. Bake for 10-15 minutes more at 350° F. until crust is done and cheese is melted.

1 serving = 312 calories, 4 meats, 2 breads
Protein: 19 gm., Fat: 10 gm., Carbohydrates: 33 gm.

Tempeh Stuffed Eggplant

Two servings

This is a tasty introduction to tempeh. Add parmesan cheese or mozzarella for more meat exchanges. (1 oz. cheese = 1 meat)

Cook in boiling water, covered, for 5 minutes:
     1 medium eggplant, cut in two, lengthwise

Drain. Scoop out the insides leaving a half inch shell. Dice the cooked pulp.

Preheat the oven to 375° F.

Simmer together for 5 minutes:
     the diced eggplant   4 oz. tempeh, diced or grated
     1 stalk celery, diced   2 tsp. tamari
     ¼ cup chopped onion   ½ cup water
     1 cup alfalfa sprouts

Remove from heat and add:
     ½ cup oatmeal
     ½ to 1 cup water

Fill eggplant halves evenly. Bake about 30 minutes.

1 serving = 317 calories, 2 meats, 1 bread, 2 vegetables
Protein: 20 gm., Fat: 7 gm., Carbohydrates: 45 gm.

Soybean-Mushroom Pilaf
Four servings

Have ready and warmed:
     3 cups cooked rice
     1½ cups cooked soybeans

Simmer until greens are tender:
     2 cups chopped mushrooms   1 cup chopped kale or spinach
     ¼ cup chopped onion   2 tsp. butter
     2 Tbsp. parsley   ¼ cup water

Stir in rice and soybeans.

Add:
     1 cup walnuts, cut up
     4 oz. cheese, shredded

Cook until cheese is melted.

1 serving = 574 calories, 4 meats, 2 breads, 2 vegetables, 1 fat
Protein: 26 gm., Fat: 24 gm., Carbohydrates: 45 gm.

Soyburgers

Mash:
>   1 cup cooked soybeans

Mix with:
>   2 Tbsp brewer's or   1 cup oatmeal
>   nutritional yeast   1 Tbsp tamari

Preheat oven to 350° F.

Saute:
>   ¼ cup chopped onion   ½ tsp. basil
>   1 clove garlic, minced   1 Tbsp oil
>   ½ tsp. oregano

Add to the beans. Mix well and form 6 flat patties. Bake on ungreased cookie sheet for 10 minutes.

Turn and top with:
>   ¼ cup tomato sauce

Bake 10-15 minutes more.

1 serving of 2 patties = 315 calories, 4 meats, 2 breads, 1 fat
Protein: 14 gm., Fat: 6 gm., Carbohydrates: 41 gm.

Tempeh with Mushroom Stuffing

One serving

Here is a quick and delicious tempeh recipe.

Preheat oven to 350° F.

Simmer together:
>   2 Tbsp. tomato sauce   1 clove garlic, minced
>   ½ cup chopped mushrooms   dash pepper
>   ¼ cup chopped onions   2 Tbsp. water

Remove from heat and mix in until cheese is melted:
    2 slices whole wheat bread, crumbled
    3 Tbsp. parmesan cheese

Lay in a dish and cover with mixture:
    4 oz. piece of tempeh, sliced in half

Bake covered for 15 minutes.

1 serving = 374 calories, 4 meats, 2 breads, 2 vegs.
Protein: 33 gm., Fat: 5 gm., Carbohydrates: 50 gm.

Tempeh Parmesan

Two servings

Simmer for 10 minutes:
    1 cup mixture of chopped tomatoes, onions and peppers
    ¼ tsp. each basil and oregano
    ¼ cup water

Set aside.

Mix:
    1 slice whole wheat bread, crumbled   **3 Tbsp. parmesan**
    ¾ cup cooked rice   **2 tsp. butter**
    1 Tbsp. nutritional yeast

Place ½ of this in an 8" X 8" casserole dish.

Steam for 10 minutes:
    3 oz. tempeh

Preheat oven to 375° F.

Cut tempeh in half, then slice the halves to form 2 sandwiches.

Slice in two and place between the two halves:
    3 oz. mozzarella cheese

Arrange in casserole dish. Top with vegetable mixture, then the other half of the crumbs. Bake for 15 minutes.

1 serving = 357 calories, 4 meats, 2 breads, 1 vegetable, 1 fat
Protein: 22 gm., Fat: 11 gm., Carbohydrates: 32 gm.

Tofu Lasagne

Two servings

Cook in boiling water until tender:
> 4 oz. whole wheat or enriched lasagne noodles

Drain noodles and set aside.

Mix:
> ½ cup tomato sauce
> ½ cup steamed broccoli, finely chopped

Preheat oven to 350° F.

In a 9" X 5" loaf pan layer half the noodles with:
> 8 oz. firm tofu
> 2 oz. mozzarella cheese, grated

Top with the rest of the noodles, tomato sauce mixture and:
> 3 Tbsp. parmesan cheese

Bake until hot, about 10 minutes.

1 serving = 426 calories, 4 meats, 2 breads, 2 vegetables
Protein: 29 gm., Fat: 12 gm., Carbohydrates: 50 gm.

Tofu Macaroni and Cheese

Four servings

Cook in 4 cups boiling water until tender:
> 2 cups uncooked whole wheat or or enriched macaroni

Drain and set aside.

Preheat oven to 375° F.

Combine in a small pan:
> ¼ cup milk
> ¼ cup milk powder

Add to milk and heat slowly, stirring until melted:
> **5 oz. cheddar cheese, grated**

Mix cheese sauce with noodles.

Stir in:
> **16 oz. tofu, diced or mashed   ½ cup chopped celery leaves**
> **2 oz. unsalted peanuts**

Place in casserole dish and heat for 5-10 minutes.

1 serving = 488 calories, 4 meats, 2 breads, 1 fat
Protein: 31 gm., Fat: 16 gm., Carbohydrates: 39 gm.

Sesame Tofu

Two servings

For non-stick pan, eliminate butter, eliminate 2 fats.

Mix together in a small bowl:
> **1 egg**
> **1 tsp. tamari**
> **1 Tbsp. water**

In another bowl combine:
> **¼ cup sesame seed**
> **¼ cup wheat germ**

Slice into 6 slices:
> **12 ozs. tofu**

Dip each slice into the egg then into the dry mixture.

Fry 3 slices at a time in:
> **2 tsp. butter**

Serve with rice or another grain or in a sandwich with lettuce and tomato.

1 serving = 395 calories, 4 meats, 3 fats
Protein: 24 gm., Fat: 16 gm., Carbohydrates: 15 gm.

Millet & Mushrooms

Four servings

I like to use different kinds of salt-free bouillon to add to the cooking water for the millet. At a health food store you can get carrot, onion, celery or mixed vegetable flavors. For non-stick pan, eliminate 1 tsp. butter and eliminate ½ fat exchange.

Cook in top of double boiler for about 15 minutes:

1 cup uncooked millet	½ cup chopped scallions
4 cups water	2 Tbsp. minced parsley
a clove minced garlic	

Place in bottom of double boiler and continue cooking 45 minutes or until liquid is absorbed.

Preheat oven to 350° F.

Add:
    1 cup chopped mushrooms
    1 tsp. butter

Beat in:
    2 eggs
    9 oz. tofu, diced

Grease an 8″ x 8″ casserole dish with:
    1 tsp. butter

Bake covered for 20-25 minutes.

1 serving = 210 calories, 2 ½ meats, 2 breads, ½ fat
Protein: 11 gm., Fat: 6 gm., Carbohydrates: 24 gm.

Mediterranean Broccoli and Rice

Four servings

Crumble into a small pan and toast:
    2 slices whole wheat bread
    1 tsp. butter

Set aside.

Simmer together over low heat for 45 minutes:
  1 cup uncooked brown rice   ½ tsp. oregano
  3 cups water   ½ tsp. kelp
  ¼ tsp. each pepper, bay,   ½ cup chopped onion
    basil and tarragon

Mix in:
  12 oz. tofu, mashed   1 pkg. frozen chopped
  2 Tbsp. nutritional yeast   broccoli, cooked

Place mixture in an ungreased 8" X 8" casserole dish and top with:
  4 oz. cheese, grated
  the toasted bread crumbs

Heat in the oven for a few minutes to melt cheese.

1 serving = 374 calories, 4 meats, 2 breads
Protein: 21 gm., Fat: 11 gm., Carbohydrates: 42 gm.

VEGETABLES

Millet with Peas and Sesame
Two servings

See photo on the cover.

Simmer over low heat until liquid is absorbed:
  ½ cup uncooked millet   ½ cup chopped onion
  2 cups water   1 tsp. salt-free bouillon

Toast in a dry skillet for a few minutes to lightly brown:
  ¼ cup sesame seeds

Mix into the cooked millet:
  1 cup cooked fresh or blanched frozen peas
  the toasted sesame seeds

1 serving = 295 calories, 3 meats, 2 breads
Protein: 11 gm., Fat: 3 gm., Carbohydrates: 40 gm.

Blender Potato Bake

Four servings

This tastes like a giant potato pancake. For non-stick pan, eliminate oil, eliminate ½ fat from exchange.

Blend in a food processor or blender:
   6 medium potatoes, diced (3 cups)   1 clove garlic, minced
   2 medium carrots, diced (1 cup)   2 eggs
   1 medium onion, chopped

Preheat oven to 350° F.

Mix blended ingredients in a bowl with:
   1 slice whole wheat bread, crumbled

Sprinkle in and stir throroughly:
   ¾ cup milk powder

Oil an 8" x 8" casserole dish with:
   1 Tbsp. of oil

Place mixture in casserole dish. Bake covered for 35 minutes. Remove from oven.

Top with:
   3 oz. grated cheddar or Swiss cheese

Return to oven and bake 5 more minutes.

1 serving = 452 calories, 4 meats, 2 breads, 1 fat
Protein: 20 gm., Fat: 10 gm., Carbohydrates: 64 gm.

Oven Eggplant

Two servings

Cook in boiling water, covered, for 5 minutes:
   1 medium eggplant

Drain and cut in two, lengthwise. Scoop out the insides leaving a half inch shell.

Mash eggplant with:

½ cup cottage cheese (low-fat)	1 tsp. basil
2 Tbsp. chopped onion	1 tsp. oregano
1 tsp. bay leaves, ground	2 Tbsp. tomato sauce

Preheat oven to 350° F.

Stuff eggplant halves, place in casserole and bake covered for 15 minutes. Add a little water to the bottom of the dish to keep eggplant moist.

Top with:
wheat germ
2 oz. provolone cheese

Bake 5 more minutes, uncovered.

1 serving = 244 calories, 2 meats, 1 bread, 2 vegetables
Protein: 10 gm., Fat: 4 gm., Carbohydrates: 10 gm.

Sweet Potatoes and Broccoli
One serving

Cook in covered sauce pan until almost done:
1 medium sweet potato or yam, diced (1 cup)
½ cup water

Add and cook until tender:
1 cup chopped fresh broccoli
additional water to cook, if necessary

Toss in with vegetables until hot:
½ cup cottage cheese (low-fat)
1 Tbsp. sesame seeds

1 Serving = 362 calories, 2 meats, 2 vegetables, 2 breads, 1 fat
Protein: 22 gm., Fat: 4 gm., Carbohydrates: 48 gm.

Sweet Potato Rice

Two servings

Cook over low heat for 40 minutes:
   ⅔ cup raw rice
   2 cups water

Stir in and heat throroughly:

2 Tbsp. chopped parsley	¼ tsp. pepper
¼ tsp. sage	¼ cup wheat germ
½ cup cooked sweet potato, mashed	1 Tbsp. brewer's or nutritional yeast

If desired, serve warm or cold with:
   4 oz. of yogurt (add 50 calories and ½ milk exchange)

1 serving = 272 calories, 3 meats, 2 breads, ½ fat
Protein: 9 gm., Fat: 2 gm., Carbohydrates: 55 gm.

Potato-Sesame Puff

3-4 servings

For non-stick pan, eliminate butter, eliminate ½ fat.

Steam until almost done:
   2 cups diced potatoes (with skins)
   1 cup fresh peas (if 1 cup frozen peas are substituted, they need not be cooked)

Preheat oven to 350° F.

Mix in:

2 Tbsp. chopped onion	2 eggs
1 Tbsp. chopped parsley	⅓ cup parmesan cheese
1 tsp. butter	2 Tbsp. sesame seed
1 cup cottage cheese (low-fat)	

Place in a buttered 8″ X 8″ casserole and top with:
   3 Tbsp. parmesan cheese
   1 Tbsp. sesame seed

Bake uncovered for 30 minutes.

1 serving = 345 calories, 2 meats, 1 ½ breads, 1 fat or 1 serving = 363 calories, 3 meats, 2 breads, ½ fat
Protein: 24 gm., Fat: 8 gm., Carbohydrates: 26 gm.

NUTS

Herbed Variety Nut Loaf

Four servings

I usually leave the sunflower seeds unground. They seem to stay the crunchiest and really add to the loaf. For non-stick pan, eliminate oil, eliminate ½ fat.

Grind in a blender:
   ½ cup cashews
   ½ cup almonds
   ½ cup peanuts

Set ground nuts aside and blend:
   1 egg
   ½ cup water
   1 cup chopped onion

Preheat oven to 350° F.

In a bowl combine the nuts and blended ingredients with:
   ⅔ cup sunflower seeds   **½ tsp. sage**
   1 cup cooked brown rice   **½ tsp. thyme**
   ⅓ cup oatmeal   **2 Tbsp. brewer's or nutritional**
   ½ cup wheat germ   **yeast**

Place mixture in an 8″ x 8″ casserole which has been greased with:
   1 Tbsp. oil

Bake uncovered for 20 minutes.

For last 3 minutes of baking top with:
   ¼ oz. grated cheese

1 serving = 659 calories, 3 meats, 1 fat, 2 breads
Protein: 26 gm., Fat: 15 gm., Carbohydrates: 45 gm.

Peanut Loaf

Four servings

This is one for peanut fans. It is good topped with yogurt. (½ cup yogurt for each serving; add ½ milk exchange). For non-stick pan, eliminate oil, eliminate ½ fat exchange.

Have ready:
    1 stalk celery, chopped
    ½ pepper, chopped
    ½ green onion, chopped

Preheat oven to 350° F.

Grind in a blender:
    1 cup peanuts
    ½ cup soy nuts

Combine blended nuts in a bowl with:
    2 Tbsp. nutritional yeast   ⅓ cup oats
    ½ cup wheat germ   ½ cup sesame seeds
    1 cup cooked brown rice

Mix in:
    The chopped vegetables
    1 egg
    1 Tbsp. tamari sauce

Place mixture in an 8″ x 8″ casserole dish which has been greased with:
    1 Tbsp. oil

Bake uncovered for 10-15 minutes.

1 serving = 530 calories, 4 meats, 2 breads, 1 ½ fats
Protein: 23 gm., Fat: 18 gm., Carbohydrates: 37 gm.

Sprouts Almondine

Four servings

Here is a chance to use your sprouts in a casserole made especially for them.

Preheat oven to 350° F.

Saute:

½ cup chopped onion	1 ½ cups chopped mushrooms
½ cup chopped celery	1 Tbsp. oil

Mix with:

1 cup almonds, ground or slivered	2 cups cooked barley
	½ tsp. bay leaves, ground
1 cup alfalfa sprouts	½ tsp. basil

Bake in an covered, ungreased 8″ x 8″ casserole dish for 30 minutes.

1 serving = 371 calories, 3 meats, 2 breads, 1 fat
Protein: 12 gm., Fat: 9 gm., Carbohydrates: 34 gm.

Cashew Stuffing

Nine servings

This loaf reminds me of a bread stuffing, but with the protein built right in. For non-stick pan, eliminate oil, eliminate ½ fat.

Have ready:
6 slices whole wheat bread, crumbled
3 cups cashews, ground

Preheat oven to 350° F.

Mix above ingredients together in order given with:

3 Tbsp. brewer's or nutritional yeast	½ tsp. marjoram
	½ tsp. oregano
3 Tbsp. parsley, chopped	2 cups chopped onion
½ tsp. sage	1 ½ cups milk (low-fat)
½ tsp. basil	3 eggs

Place in a 9″ x 13″ casserole which has been greased with:
1 Tbsp. oil

Bake for 35-40 minutes.

1 serving = 374 calories, 3 meats, 2 breads, 1 fat
Protein: 14 gm., Fat: 8 gm., Carbohydrates: 26 gm.

Elbow Macaroni with Cashew "Cheese"

Two servings

This really does taste similar to macaroni and cheese, but without the animal fat and the recipe can easily be doubled to serve four.

Cook in boiling water (salted if not on a salt-free diet):
　　2 cups cooked whole wheat or enriched elbow macaroni

Drain and set aside.

Sauce

Blend to a fine powder in the blender:
　　½ cup cashews

Add and blend again:
　　½ pepper, chopped
　　½ onion, chopped
　　2 Tbsp. brewer's yeast
　　2 Tbsp. lemon juice
　　1 clove garlic, minced
　　1 ½ cups water

Topping

Mix together in a small saucepan:
　　¼ cup mixture of bran and wheat germ
　　1 Tbsp. brewer's or nutritional yeast
　　1 tsp. butter
　　1 Tbsp. parsley

Saute until hot, but not browned.

Preheat oven to 350° F.

Place sauce in a pan with the cooked macaroni. Stir and heat until thick. Pour into an 8" X 8" ungreased casserole dish and bake for 10 minutes. Top with topping and return to oven for 5 more minutes.

1 serving = 439 calories, 4 meats, 2 breads, ½ fat
Protein: 18 gm., Fat: 6 gm., Carbohydrates: 52 gm.

CHEESE & EGGS

Buckwheat-Millet Special

Four servings

Simmer together for 20 minutes:
½ cup uncooked buckwheat	4 cups water
½ cup uncooked millet	½ cup chopped onions

Preheat oven to 350° F.

Beat in:
1 cup cottage cheese	1 cup grated carrots
2 eggs	4 tsp. sesame tahini
½ cup peanut butter	

Bake in ungreased 8" x 8" casserole dish for 15-20 minutes.

1 serving = 251 calories, 4 meats, 2 breads
Protein: 15 gm., Fat: 11 gm., Carbohydrates: 26 gm.

Baked Egg Patties

Two servings

Preheat oven to 350° F.

Mix together in the order given:
4 hard cooked eggs, chopped	1 Tbsp. chives
2 cups cooked brown rice	2 Tbsp. water
½ cup chopped onion	2 Tbsp. mayonnaise

Shape into 12 patties and coat each with:
    ½ cup wheat germ

Bake on ungreased baking sheet for 15 minutes.

1 serving of six = 425 calories, 2 ½ meats, 2 breads, 2 fats
Protein: 25 gm., Fat: 17 gm., Carbohydrates: 58 gm.

Broccoli & Swiss

Four servings

Cauliflower, green beans, zucchini or other non-starch vegetables can be used here in place of the broccoli. For non-stick pan, eliminate oil, eliminate ½ fat.

Toast by heating in dry pan until crisp, but not brown:
 ½ cup sunflower seeds

Steam lightly, drain and chop finely:
 2 cups broccoli

Preheat oven to 325° F.

Mix broccoli with:
 1 cup chopped mushrooms   ½ cup wheat germ
 ½ cup chopped onion   2 cups oatmeal
 ½ cup grated Swiss cheese   the toasted sesame seeds
 2 eggs

Place mixture in an 8″ x 8″ casserole which has been greased with:
 1 Tbsp. oil

Bake covered for 20-25 minutes.

1 serving = 586 calories, 4 meats, 2 breads, 1 fat
Protein: 29 gm., Fat: 15 gm., Carbohydrates: 65 gm.

Millet Cottage Cheese Casserole

Four servings

This is one of my favorites. I like to add a vegetable, broccoli, green beans or carrots are favorites. Be sure to count each half cup of them per serving as a vegetable exchange. For non-stick pans, eliminate butter and eliminate one fat exchange.

Simmer for 20 minutes:
 ½ cup millet   1 tsp. instant, salt-free
 2 cups water   vegetable bouillon

Preheat oven to 325° F.

Stir in:
⅓ cup finely chopped celery	2 eggs, lightly beaten
	1 cup cottage cheese

Place mixture in a one quart casserole which has been greased with:
2 tsp. butter

Bake covered for about 20 minutes until firm, but not browned.

1 serving = 160 calories, 2 breads, 3 meats, 1 fat
Protein: 11 gm., Fat: 5 gm., Carbohydrates: 12 gm.

Cheese Lasagne

Three servings

Cook in boiling water until tender:
6 oz. whole wheat or enriched lasagne noodles

Drain noodles and set aside.

Combine:
½ cup tomato sauce
1 cup mixture of onions, peppers & mushrooms, chopped

Mix in a separate bowl:
1 ½ cups cottage cheese (low fat)	2 eggs
	1 Tbsp. parmesan cheese

Preheat oven to 350° F.

In an 8" X 8" casserole layer half the noodles, the cottage cheese mixture and:
3 oz. mozzarella cheese, grated

Top with tomato sauce mix and the rest of the noodles.

Sprinkle with:
2 Tbsp. parmesan cheese

Bake for 25 minutes.

1 serving = 500 calories, 4 meats, 2 breads, 1 fat
Protein: 36 gm., Fat: 10 gm., Carbohydrates: 52 gm.

Mushroom Supper Cake

Two servings

This is a very filling supper, served with a salad and vegetables.

Simmer in a covered frying pan for 10 minutes:

1 cup chopped mushrooms	1 clove garlic, minced
½ cup chopped peppers & onions	1 tsp. butter
	1 Tbsp. water

Remove from heat and mix in:
    4 slices whole wheat bread, crumbled

Allow bread to soak up flavors for 10 minutes.

Preheat oven to 350° F.

Beat in:
    2 eggs
    3 Tbsp. parmesan cheese
    ¾ cup cottage cheese (low fat)

Bake for 15 minutes in an ungreased shallow dish.

Sprinkle on:
    2 oz. Swiss cheese, grated

Return to the oven and bake 5 more minutes.

1 serving = 478 calories, 4 meats, 2 breads, 1 fat
Protein: 33 gm., Fat: 13 gm., Carbohydrates: 31 gm.

Spinach, Cheese and Rice Bake

Four servings

You can use another non-starchy vegetable in place of spinach for variety. Or try using more than one; zucchini, peppers, and mushrooms, for example. For a non-stick pan, eliminate 1 Tbsp. butter and eliminate ½ fat exchange.

Simmer for about 20 minutes or until liquid is absorbed:
- **1 cup uncooked brown rice**
- **2 cups water**
- **½ cup chopped onion**
- **1 clove garlic, minced**

Cube or grate into the cooked rice:
- **3 oz. Swiss cheese**

Stir until melted evenly.

Add:
- **2 cups shredded spinach**
- **2 eggs**
- **½ cup milk (low-fat)**

Preheat oven to 350° F.

Grease an 8″ X 8″ casserole dish with:
- **1 Tbsp. butter**

Place mixture in dish. Melt in a small pan:
- **2 Tbsp. butter**

Mix in:
- **½ cup wheat germ**
- **1 Tbsp. parsley**
- **1 ½ Tbsp. parmesan cheese**

Spread this on top of casserole. Bake uncovered for 20 minutes.

1 serving = 409 calories, 3 meats, 2 breads, 1 fat
Protein: 19 gm., Fat: 13 gm., Carbohydrates: 40 gm.

Crepes with Three Great Fillings

Makes two crepes

Crepe Batter:

Mix together in order
    ½ cup whole wheat flour   2 eggs
    ¼ cup wheat germ or cornmeal   1 Tbsp. oil
    1 cup milk (low-fat)

Use about 2 tablespoons of batter for each crepe, rotating pan to thin batter to about 6-7 inches in diameter. Turn once. These come out best when made on a non-stick pan.

2 crepes = 355 calories, 2 bread, 1 fat; or 1 bread, ½ milk, 1 fat
Protein: 16 gm., Fat: 12 gm., Carbohydrates: 39 gm.

Tofu-Ratatouille Filling

Simmer until tender:
    1 small eggplant, diced finely   2 Tbsp. tomato sauce
    ¼ cup chopped onion   ¼ cup water
    ¼ cup chopped pepper

Stir in:
    oz. tofu, diced or crumbled

Preheat oven to 350° F.

Divide between four crepes. Roll crepes up with filling inside.

Top with:
    4 oz. mozzarella cheese, shredded

You can also add cheese to filling. Heat about 10 minutes to melt cheese.

2 fillings = 405 calories, 3 meats, 2 vegetables
Protein: 32 gm., Fat: 18 gm., Carbohydrates: 19 gm.

Cottage Cheese Filling

Mix together:
  2 cups cottage cheese (low-fat)
  1 cup alfalfa sprouts
  ½ cup scallions, chopped
  1 tsp. dried tarragon

Fill four crepes evenly. Serve hot or cold.

2 fillings = 254 calories, 2 meats, ½ vegetable
Protein: 30 gm., Fat: 6 gm., Carbohydrates: 12 gm.

Nutty Cabbage-Slaw Filling

Have ready:
  1 cup plain yogurt

Toss together and soak for at least 1 hour:
  2 cups finely shredded cabbage   ¼ cup cider vinegar
  ¼ cup chopped onion   1 tsp. dill weed
  ¼ cup chopped green pepper   2 tsp. caraway seed
  1 cup carrots, grated   ½ tsp. black pepper

Mix in:
  24 walnut halves, chopped finely

Fill four crepes. Serve hot or cold.

Top each crepe with:
  ¼ cup yogurt.

Filling for 2 crepes = 188 calories, ½ meat, ½ milk, 1 fat, 1 vegetable
Protein: 9 gm., Fat: 16 gm., Carbohydrates: 19 gm.

BEANS

It's a good idea to cook up some beans whenever you have the time, so you will have them for preparing a quick meal. Cooked beans will last about a week in the refrigerator, or can be frozen in measured portions. Many of the recipes in this section are also good to take along cold for lunch.

Patty's Garbanzo Patties

Four servings

For non-stick pan, eliminate oil, eliminate 1 fat.

Have ready:
　　2 cups cooked garbanzo beans

Grind in a food processor or blender:
　　1 cup garbanzo beans

Remove and set aside.

Blend:
　　1 egg　　　　　　　　　½ cup chopped onions
　　2 Tbsp. tomato sauce　　1 clove garlic, crushed

Mix with ground beans.

Combine with:
　　1 cup whole garbazo beans　　⅓ cup oatmeal
　　1 cup chopped mushrooms　　⅓ cup rolled wheat or oats
　　4 slices whole wheat　　　　1 Tbsp. brewer's or nutritional
　　　bread, crumbled　　　　　　yeast
　　⅓ cup sesame seeds

Let sit ten minutes so grains can absorb some liquid.

Form eight patties and fry four at a time in:
　　1 Tbsp.oil

1 serving of two patties = 491 calories, 3 meats, 2 breads, 1 fat
Protein: 21 gm., Fat: 11 gm., Carbohydrates: 63 gm.

Corny-Crunchy Garbanzos

Two servings

Cook over low heat for 30 minutes:

⅓ cup uncooked brown rice	½ tsp. rosemary
1 cup water	1 clove garlic, chopped
¼ tsp. sage	2 Tbsp. parsley
¼ tsp. thyme	½ cup chopped onion

Stir in and heat:
    ½ cup frozen corn
    1 cup cooked garbanzo beans

For topping, heat in pan:
    3 Tbsp. sesame seeds
    ¼ cup wheat germ
    2 tsp. butter

Mix until seeds and wheat germ are coated with butter. Sprinkle topping over the beans and rice.

1 serving = 574 calories, 4 meats, 2 breads, 1 fat
Protein: 24 gm., Fat: 6 gm., Carbohydrates: 73 gm.

Three-Bean Delight

Four servings

Toss together:

1 cup cooked kidney beans	1 cup chopped onion
1 cup cooked garbanzo beans	½ cup chopped green pepper
1 cup cooked lima beans	4 tsp. olive oil

Serve hot or cold, with a grain or bread or dairy product to compliment protein. To serve cold for a salad add a few drops of lemon juice or vinegar.

1 serving = 260 calories, 2½ meats, 2 vegetables, 1 fat
Protein: 14 gm., Fat: 1 gm., Carbohydrates: 42 gm.

Hearty Beans and Rice Supper

Four servings

Simmer over low heat for 35 minutes:

2/3 cup uncooked brown rice   1/2 cup chopped green pepper
1 1/2 cups water   1/2 tsp bay leaves, ground
1 cup chopped celery   1/2 tsp. basil
1/2 cup chopped onion   1/2 tsp. oregano

Mix in and cook 10 minutes:

2 cups cooked pinto beans   2 fresh tomatoes, chopped
1 cup fresh or frozen corn   1 tsp. olive oil

Serve with a sprinkling of:

2 oz. grated cheddar cheese

1 serving = 320 calories, 2 meats, 2 breads, 1 vegetable
Protein: 16 gm., Fat: 4 gm., Carbohydrates: 55 gm.

Kidney Bean Pie

Four servings

Crust

Preheat oven to 350° F.

Mix together:

1 1/2 cups cornmeal   1 egg
1 cup cottage cheese   1/4 cup water

Press into a pie plate which has been oiled with:

1 Tbsp. oil

Bake crust alone for 10 minutes.

Filling

Heat:
    2 ½ cups cooked kidney beans   ¼ cup chopped mix of
    ¼ cup tomato sauce   onions and peppers

Pour bean mixture into crust and bake for 10 minutes more at 350°F.

1 serving = 427 calories, 4 meats, 2 breads
Protein: 22 gm., Fat: 8 gm., Carbohydrates: 64 gm.

Basic Bean Loaf

Four servings

This loaf is good topped with yogurt. I use about ½ cup yogurt for each serving. Add ½ milk exchange.

Have ready:
    2 slices whole wheat bread, crumbled
    2 cups cooked pinto beans
    ½ cup ground peanuts
    ½ cup chopped celery
    ½ cup chopped onion

Preheat oven to 350° F.

Mix above ingredients together with:
    ⅔ cup oatmeal
    1 egg
    ½ cup water

Place mixture in a small loaf pan or an 8″ X 8″ casserole which has been greased with:
    1 Tbsp. oil

Bake covered for 20-25 minutes.

1 serving = 394 calories, 2 breads, 3 meats, 1 fat
Protein: 19 gm., Fat: 9 gm., Carbohydrates: 49 gm.

Pintos with Cornbread Topping

Four servings

You can try reversing this and using the topping on the bottom and the beans on top. Either way it's great!

Simmer over medium heat for 10 minutes:
- 3 cups cooked pinto beans
- ⅓ cup tomato sauce
- ⅓ cup chopped onion
- ⅓ cup chopped green pepper

Preheat oven to 400° F.

For topping, mix in a small bowl:
- 4 tsp. butter, melted
- 1 cup cornmeal
- 1 cup milk (low-fat)
- 1 tsp. chili powder (optional)

Put beans in an 8" x 8" dish, then pour cornmeal mixture on top and bake for 15-20 minutes, uncovered.

1 serving = 376 calories, 2 ½ meats, 2 breads, 1 fat
Protein: 16 gm., Fat: 4 gm., Carbohydrates: 60 gm.

Pasta I Fagoli

One serving

This recipe can easily be doubled or quadrupled.

Boil until tender (about 10 minutes):
- ½ cup whole wheat or enriched elbow macaroni
- 1 cup water

Saute until tender:
- 1 Tbsp. chopped onion
- 1 tsp. olive oil

Pintos with Cornbread Topping, this page

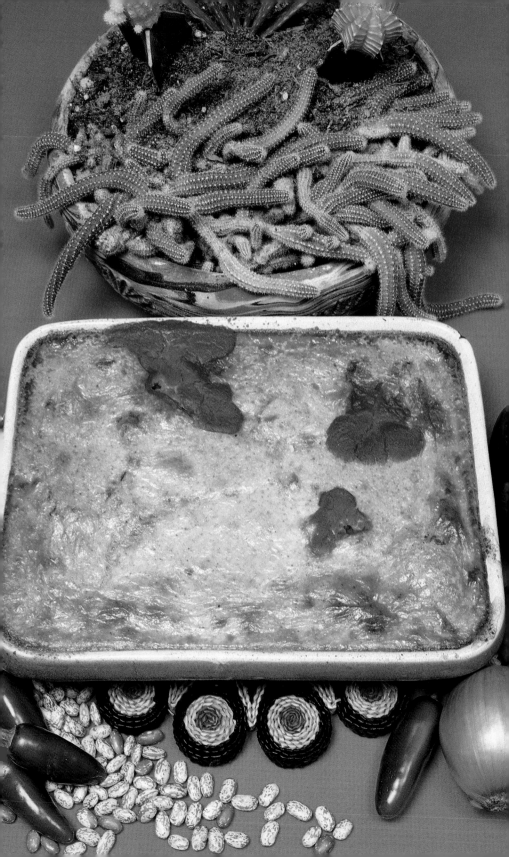

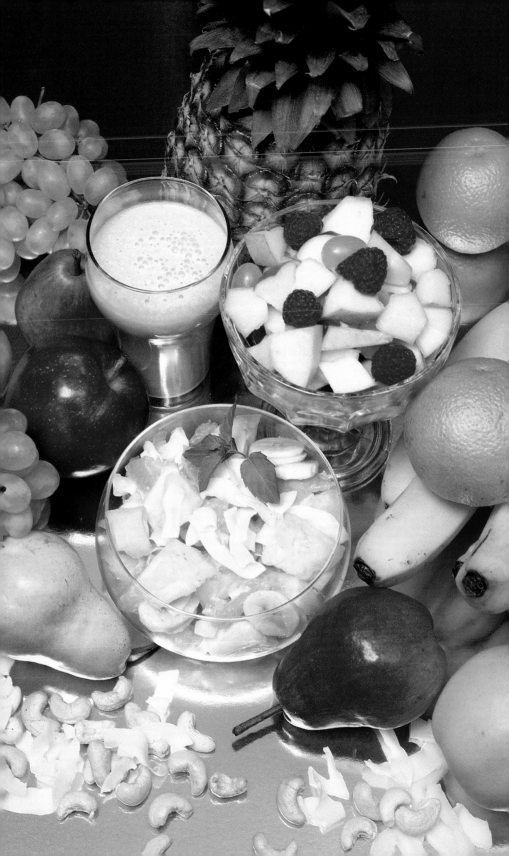

Add and simmer:
  1 Tbsp. tomato sauce
  ½ cup pinto beans, cooked
  2 Tbsp. sesame seeds
  2 Tbsp. parmesan cheese

Stir in macaroni.

1 serving = 404 calories, 3 meats, 2 breads, 1 fat
Protein: 21 gm., Fat: 5 gm., Carbohydrates: 51 gm.

Walnut-Lentil Loaf

Nine servings

An ounce of Swiss cheese on each serving adds one meat exchange and combines nicely with the walnuts and lentils. Curry powder to taste can be used in place of thyme, basil and oregano.

Have ready:
  1 slice whole wheat bread,   ½ cup chopped walnuts
    crumbled   ½ cup chopped onion
  2 cups cooked lentils

Preheat oven to 350° F.

Mix together above ingredients in order given with:
  ½ cup wheat germ   2 eggs
  2 Tbsp. sesame seeds   ½ cup water
  ½ tsp. thyme   1 Tbsp. vinegar
  ¼ tsp. basil   2 Tbsp. brewer's or nutritional
  ¼ tsp. oregano   yeast

Place mixture in a small loaf or in a 8″ X 8″ dish which has been greased with:
  1 Tbsp. oil

Bake for 35-40 minutes.

1 serving = 168 calories, 3 meats, 2 breads, 1 fat
Protein: 9 gm., Fat: 6 gm., Carbohydrates: 15 gm.

Tropical Fruit Salad, p.124, Northern Fruit Salad, p.125, Creamy Peanut and Pineapple Shake, p.53

Falafel

Four servings

Preheat oven to 350° F.

Grind in a food processor or blender:

3 cups cooked garbanzo beans	1 Tbsp. lemon juice
	½ cup chopped onion

Remove and mix with:

2 Tbsp. whole wheat pastry flour	¼ cup sesame seed
¼ cup wheat germ	¼ tsp. pepper
¼ cup parsley	¼ tsp. garlic powder

Form into 20 falafel balls.

Heat in a large baking dish in the oven:
   2 Tbsp. oil

Place falafel in the dish and bake 15 minutes, stirring occasionally.

1 serving of 5 falafels = 434 calories, 3 meats, 2 breads, 1 fat
Protein: 20 gm., Fat: 9 gm., Carbohydrates: 56 gm.

Grainburgers

Eight patties

For non-stick pan, eliminate oil and all fat exchanges.

Simmer together until liquid is absorbed:

⅔ cup uncooked brown rice	⅓ cup chopped green pepper
2 cups water	1 tsp. vegetable bouillon
⅓ cup chopped celery	
⅓ cup chopped onion	
(salt and sugar free)	

Add:

1 egg	⅓ cup wheat germ
⅓ cup cornmeal	⅓ cup oatmeal

Form eight patties. Brown four at a time in:
   1½ Tbsp. oil

1 serving of 3 patties = 318 calories, 2 breads, 3 meats, 2 fats
Protein: 11 gm., Fat: 11 gm., Carbohydrates: 52 gm.

Snacks

If you can make your snacks interesting and different, you will be less tempted to eat something you shouldn't, like potato chips or packaged cookies. Don't think of it as something you just want to get over with because you have to eat at a certain time. Take your time and make it enjoyable!

Quick Rice Pudding

Two servings

Preheat oven to 350° F.

Mix together in order given:
    1 cup cooked brown rice
    ½ cup milk (low-fat)
    1 egg, beaten
    1½ Tbsp. raisins

Pour into a small casserole dish. Place this dish in another oven-proof dish containing an inch or two of water.

Sprinkle with:
    1 tsp. nutmeg

Bake for 20-30 minutes.

1 serving = 178 calories, 1 bread, 1 fruit, 1 milk
Protein: 7 gm., Fat: 2 gm., Carbohydrates: 28 gm.

Tropical Fruit Salad

Four servings

See photo, page 120.

Toss together:
    4 fresh apricots or oranges, pitted & cut up
    1 cup diced fresh pineapple
    1 banana, sliced
    4 Tbsp. unsweetened coconut
    2 tsp. lemon juice

Serve.

1 serving = 97 calories, 2 fruits
Protein: 1 gm., Fat: 2 gm., Carbohydrates: 16 gm.

Banana Split

One serving

Split in half lengthwise:
   1 banana

Top in order given with:
   ½ cup yogurt (low-fat)
   6 walnuts, chopped
   2 Tbsp. wheat germ

256 calories, 2 fruits, 1 fat, ½ milk, 1.2 bread; or 2 fruits, 1 fat, 1 milk
Protein: 11 gm., Fat: 8 gm., Carbohydrates: 40 gm.

Northern Fruit Salad

Four servings

See photo, page 120.

Toss together:
   2 medium apples, diced
   2 medium pears, diced
   10 cherries, pitted, or raspberries
   10 grapes
   2 tsp. lemon juice

Serve.

1 serving = 110 calories, 2 fruits
Protein: 0 gm., Fat: 0 gm., Carbohydrates: 28 gm.

Nut Mix

One serving

Mix together:
   6 walnuts
   1½ oz. cashews
   1 tsp. sunflower seeds
   1½ Tbsp. raisins

Serve.

1 serving = 260 calories, 3 fats, 2 fruits
Protein: 8 gm., Fat: 6 gm., Carbohydrates: 22 gm.

Banchew Shake

One serving

Blend to a fine powder:
    2 oz. cashews

Remove and blend:
    ½ cup milk
    ½ banana
    1 tsp. vanilla (optional)

Add cashews and blend again at high speed.

427 calories, 1 milk, 2 fats; or 1 fruit, ½ milk, 4 fats
Protein: 14 gm., Fat: 7 gm., Carbohydrates: 36 gm.

The Islander

One serving

See photo on the cover.

Scoop out seeds from:
    ½ cantaloupe

Top with:
    ½ cup yogurt
    ¼ cup unsweetened coconut, grated
    10 almonds, chopped or sliced

318 calories, 2 fruits, ½ milk, 2 fats
Protein: 10 gm., Fat: 11 gm., Carbohydrates: 32 gm.

The Winter Warmer

One serving

Preheat oven to 375° F.

Place in small casserole dish:
    1 cup diced potatoes

Add:

    1 Tbsp. water   ¼ tsp. each dill, oregano

    1 Tbsp. cider vinegar   ⅛ tsp. pepper

Stir to coat potatoes. Cover dish and bake for 20 minutes.

1 serving = 114 calories, 1½ breads
Protein: 3 gm., Fat: 0 gm., Carbohydrates: 26 gm.

Popcorn

One serving

See photo on the back cover.

This is a good snack for a diabetic person because of the large, satisfying quantity that is allowed for 1 bread. Without butter or salt, it is low in calories and provides good roughage and some trace minerals. Here are some other ingredients which can be added to popcorn to create new snack ideas. (⅓ cup unpopped will equal 3 cups popped for 69 calories and 1 bread exchange)

To 3 cups of popcorn:
Mix in:

    1½ Tbsp. peanuts

    1½ Tbsp. raisins

249 calories, 1 bread, 2 fats, 2 fruits
Protein: 10 gm., Fat: 3 gm., Carbohydrates: 47 gm.

Mix in:

    3 Tbsp. parmesan cheese

    1½ Tbsp. peanuts

228 calories, 1 bread, 2 fats, ½ milk
Protein: 12 gm., Fat: 5 gm., Carbohydrates: 25 gm.

Sprinkle on:

    1 Tbsp. brewer's or nutritional yeast

This is really a unique and tasty combination.

92 calories, 1 bread
Protein: 3 gm., Fat: 0 gm., Carbohydrates: 16 gm.

Mix in:

    ½ cup low-fat cottage cheese

169 calories, 1½ meats; or 1 bread, 1 milk
Protein: 16 gm., Fat: 3 gm., Carbohydrates: 19 gm.

The Energizer

Toss together:
    1 Tbsp. cashews
    1 Tbsp. sunflower seeds
    2 Tbsp. wheat germ
    ½ cup oatmeal
    2 tsp. chopped dates

Put in a dessert bowl:
    ½ cup yogurt

Top with:
    the nut mixture
    ½ banana, sliced

1 serving = 620 calories, 2 breads, ½ milk, 3 fats, 2 fruit
Protein: 23 gm., Fat: 11 gm., Carbohydrates: 97 gm.

Nine P.M. Rescue

Mix:
    ½ apple, diced finely
    1 Tbsp. peanut butter

Spread on:
    1 slice whole wheat bread

Top with:
    1 oz. cheddar cheese, sliced

Heat in the oven.

250 calories, 2 fats, ½ fruit; or 1 meat, 1 bread 1 milk, ½ fruit
Protein: 10 gm., Fat: 6 gm., Carbohydrates: 22 gm.

Yogurt

Yogurt is easy to make, and the homemade kind is always fresh.
You can double or triple this recipe according to your needs.

Mix in the top of a double boiler:
   4 cups fresh low-fat milk
   ⅓ cup powdered (non-instant) milk

Use an egg beater or an electric mixer to make it smooth.
Heat milk up to 180°, using a candy thermometer to test the
temperature. Remove from heat and allow to cool down to 120°.

While milk is cooling, fill with hot water:
   2 pint jars

Be sure to keep everything clean.

Put into a cup and leave at room temperature while the milk is
cooling:
   2 Tbsp. yogurt (be sure to get a brand with active cultures)

   Get out a styrofoam or plastic ice chest and place a large bowl with
cover inside. When the milk is cool enough, mix a small amount into
the yogurt, then add that to the rest of the milk, stirring thoroughly.
Empty the hot water out of the jars and fill them with the yogurt.
Cover the jars and place them around the bowl in the ice chest. Fill
the bowl with boiling water, cover it, and then cover the ice chest.
Incubate the yogurt 5 hours.
   When incubation time is up, remove the yogurt and place the jars
in the freezer for two hours, then remove and put into the
refrigerator. You can put the yogurt directly into the refrigerator, but
the consistency will be more even if it is cooled down first by the
colder temperature of the freezer.

Herbs

I have found these herbs to go best with these foods. You may prefer other combinations, but if you are new to experimenting with herbs, try these suggestions.

Tea
basil	fennel
cinnamon	ginger
coriander	mint
cloves	sage

Baked into Bread
anise seed	fennel
caraway seed	garlic
cardamon seed	ginger
cinnamon	parsely
cloves	

Beans
basil	oregano
bay	pepper
cumin	rosemary
curry	sage
garlic	

Lentils
basil
bay
cumin

Hard Cheese Dishes
basil	dill
bay	garlic
caraway seed	oregano
celery seed	pepper
chives	

Egg Dishes
bay	marjoram
basil	parsley
celery seed	pepper
chives	savory
dill	tarragon
fennel	

With Cottage Cheese or Yogurt
basil	marjoram
bay	parsley
chives	sage
cinnamon	thyme
dill	

In Salad Dressings
basil	garlic
bay	marjoram
caraway seed	pepper
celery seed	rosemary
chives	sage
dill	tarragon
fennel	thyme

Peas

basil	parsley
bay	rosemary
chives	thyme

Green or Wax Beans

basil	oregano
bay	savory
marjoram	thyme

Carrots

basil
bay
chives
parsley

Sweet Potato

cinnamon
parsley
pepper

Tomatoes

basil	oregano
bay	pepper
chives	tarragon
garlic	

Potatoes

basil	dill
caraway seed	parsley
chives	pepper
celery seed	thyme

Corn

basil	pepper
bay	thyme
chives	

Mustard Greens, Collards
Spinach, Kale

basil	marjoram
bay	oregano
chives	pepper
garlic	

Cabbage

basil	cumin
bay	curry
caraway seed	pepper

Zucchini or Summer Squash

basil	garlic
bay	oregano
chives	pepper
dill	tarragon

Brussel Sprouts, Broccoli,
& Cauliflower

basil
bay
chives
oregano

Glossary

Adult Onset Diabetes—A condition of insulin "resistance". Obesity can makes it even more difficult for the cells to bind and utilize insulin. Stress and heredity can also influence its development. Often, blood levels of insulin are actually elevated in this condition.

Amino Acids—These are the chemical components of protein. Of the 22 amino acids, nine cannot be produced by the body and must be supplied as part of the protein we eat.

Basal Metabolic Rate—The minimum metabolic activity required to maintain life processes such as heart beat and respiration.

Calorie—This is the measure of the potential energy or fuel value of a food.

Carbohydrates—One of the three major energy sources in food. Composed of starches and sugars, it yields about four calories per gram.

Cholesterol—A fat-like substance that is required by all the cells of the body. It is a normal component of the blood, but is of concern when present in excessive amounts. It is manufactured in the liver and is ingested in the consumption of foods of animal origin.

Dietetic—This does not mean "diabetic." It usually denotes a decrease in calories or some modification of ingredients. The calories may still exceed the acceptable limits for a diabetic. These foods usually contain artificial sweeetners.

Emulsifier—A chemical used to prevent the separation of oil and water. It is often found in salad dressings.

Fat—One of the three major energy sources in food. It yields about nine calories per gram.

Fatty Acids—These are essential acids which cannot be made by the body and must be obtained from food, mainly polyunsaturated oils.

Fiber—An indigestible part of fruits, vegetables and grains. It is important because it stimulates the gastro—intestinal tract.

Food Exchanges—Foods grouped together on a list according to similarities in food value. A single exchange of measured amounts are approximately equal in amounts of calories, carbohydrates, proteins, fats, minerals and vitamins.

Glucose—A single molecule sugar utilized for energy by the body.

Gram—A unit of mass and weight in the metric system. An ounce equals 28.4 grams.

Hydrogenated Fats— Liquid vegetable oils that have been combined with additional hydrogen to become solid, saturated fats, such as stick margarine and vegetable shortening.

Hyperglycemia—The increase of blood sugar levels due to lack of insulin or too much food. The onset is gradual and the symptoms are dry mouth, excessive thirst and urination, general ill feeling, acetone breath, and eventually, coma.

Hypoglycemia—The decrease of blood sugar levels due to too much insulin or too little food. The onset is sudden and the symptoms are moist skin, nervousness and confusion, sweating, shaking, hunger, weakness and eventually, coma.

Insulin— A hormone which clears the blood of excess sugar by delivering it to body cells where it is used for energy or converted to fat for storage.

Juvenile Onset Diabetes—This may be related to specific genetic factors including an immunologic condition in which anti-bodies form and work against the action of insulin. There is also the possibility of a type of virus infection as a cause of diabetes.

Ketoacidosis—This is the result of prolonged hyperglycemia. As the blood sugar levels increase because of lack of insulin, the body loses fluid and becomes dehydrated. Fats are broken down in an attempt to get fuel. Ketone bodies are the end products of improper fat breakdown. These accumulate in the blood then spill over into the urine. If insulin and fluids are not given soon enough, coma can result.

Mineral—A substance essential in small amounts to build and repair body tissue and/or control body functions.

Monounsaturated Fats—Fats that are predominately monounsaturated are chemically capable of absorbing additional hydrogen, but not as much hydrogen as polyunsaturated fatty acids. These fats have little effect on blood cholesterol. Examples are olive oil and peanut oil.

"Natural" Food—Ideally, foods that have been minimally processed or not processed at all. Usually they contain no artificial ingredients. however, the Food and Drug Administration's policy on the use of the word "natural" on food labels is very loose. Often, it appears on highly processed products which may only have one truly "natural" ingredient. For example, "Natural Orange Flavor" fruit drink has as its only real ingredient orange oil that is artificially extracted from oranges. The other ingredients are sugar, citric acid, malto dextrin, calcium phosphates, vitamin C, artificial flavor, cellulose and xanthan gums, artificial color, vitamin A palmitate, BHA and alpha tocopherol.

NPU (Net Protein Utilization)—The percentage of absorbed protein that the body actually uses.

Nutrient—The chemical constituents of foods that are utilized in the body: proteins, carbohydrates, fats, vitamins, minerals, water.

Nutrition—A combination of processes by which the body receives and uses the materials necessary for maintenance of functions, for energy, and for growth and renewal.

"Organic" Foods—All foods are organic chemically, since they are composed of carbon, hydrogen, oxygen and sometimes nitrogen. Foods labeled "organic" may mean that they have been grown or produced without the use of chemical fertilizer or pesticides. However, residues of chemicals are sometimes found on these products due to long-term contamination of once chemically fertilized soil or from chemicals that have leaked into the "organic" field through irrigation, road drainoffs, or even the air. There are differences from state to state in what constitutes an "organic" food and only a few states have definite laws.

Polyunsaturated Fats—Fats that are predominantly polyunsaturated are chemically capable of absorbing additional hydrogen. These fats are usually of vegetable origin, are liquid at room temperature, and tend to lower the cholesterol in the blood. Examples are safflower oil and corn oil. Also, the fat in fish is predominantly polyunsaturated.

Preservative—The generic term for substances added to food to prevent spoilage.

Protein—One of the three major nutrient groups in foods which contain amino acids that are essential for the life processes. Protein provides about four calories per gram.

Processed Foods—These are foods that have been treated in some way to inhibit deterioration and increase the shelf life of the food, (i.e. freezing, canning). Processed foods are also presweetened cereals, vitamin-enriched breakfast bars, frozen dinners, American cheese, packaged mixes and other canned, dried, forzen and preserved products.

RDA—(Recommended Dietary Allowance)—A list devised by the National Academy of Sciences of the recommended levels of seventeen essential nutrients that should be consumed to meet the nutritional needs of practically all healthy persons. This guide incorporates a safety margin to compensate for any individual differences and normal stresses of daily living.

Saturated Fats—Fats that are predominantly saturated are chemically not capable of absorbing any more hydrogen. These fats are usually of animal origin (except coconut and palm oils), are solid at room temperature, and tend to

increase the amount of cholesterol in the blood. Examples
are butter and the fat in meat and poultry.

Sweetners, artificial—Non-nutritive chemical substances used
in place of sugar to provide a sweet taste with no calories.
These include saccharin and cyclamates. The possible cancer
risks of these sweeteners makes their advantages not worth
the chance.

Vitamin—A substance that is essential in small amounts to
assist in body processes and functions.

Selective Bibliography of Books Pertaining to Vegetarianism & Diabetes

Diabetes

Addanki, Sam, *Diabetes Breakthrough: Control Through Nutrition,* 1981, Pinnacle Books.

Anderson, James W., *Diabetes: A Practical New Guide To Healthy Living,* 1981, Arco.

Anderson, James W., Ward, Kyleen; and Sieling, Beverly; *HCF Diets: A User's Guide,* Lexington: University of Kentucky Diabetes Fund, 1979.

Bennett, Margaret, *The Peripatic Diabetic,* 1969, Hawthorne Books.

Biermann, June & Toohey, Barbara, *The Diabetic's Book: All Your Questions Answered,* 1981. J.P. Tarcher.

Biermann, June & Toohey, Barbara, *The Diabetic's Sport & Exercise Book: How To Play Your Way To Better Health,* 1977, Harper-Row.

Biermann, June and Toohey, Barbara, *The Diabetic's Total Health Book,* 1982, J. P. Tarcher.

Gibbons, Euell & Joe, *Feast on a Diabetic Diet,* 1969, Fawcett Crest Books.

Krall, Leo P., ed., *Joslin Diabetes Manual,* Phildelphia: Lea & Fabiger, 1978.

Vegetarianism

Barkas, Janet, *The Vegetable Passion*, New York: Scribners, 1975
Doyle, Rodger P., *The Vegetarian Handbook: A Guide to Vegetarian Nutrition*, New York: Crown, 1979.
Hewitt, Jean, *The New York Times Natural Foods Cookbook*, New York: Quadrangle Books, 1971.
Lappe, Frances Moore, *Diet For a Small Planet*, New York: Ballantine Books, Division of Random House, 1973.
Lappe, Frances Moore, *Recipes For a Small Planet*, New York: Ballantine Books, Division of Random House, 1973.
Null, Gary, *The New Vegetarian: Building Your Health Through Natural Eating*, New York: Morrow, 1978.
Robertson, Laurel; Flinders, Carol; and Godfrey, Bronwen: *Laurel's Kitchen*, Petuluma, Calif: Nilgri Press, 1976.

General Nutrition

Ashley, Richard & Duggal, Heidi, *Dictinary of Nutrition*, New York: St. Martin's Press, 1975.
Brody, Jane, *Jane Brody's Nutrition Book*, New York, Bantam Books, by arrangement with W.W. Norton & Co., Inc. 1982.
Davis, Adele, *Let's Eat Right to Keep Fit*
Deutsch, Ronald M., *The Realities of Nutrition*, New York, Palo Alto: Bull 1976.
Goldbeck, Nikki and David, *The Supermarket Handbook*, New York: Harper & Row, 1973.
Mayer, Jean, *A Diet for Living*, New York: David McKay, 1975.
Null, Gary and Steve, *The Complete Handbook of Nutrition*, New York: Dell Publishing Co., Inc., 1972.
Nutrition Search, Inc., *Nutrition Almanac, Revised Edition*, New York: McGraw-Hill, 1979.
Tver, David F. and Russell, Percy, *The Nutrition and Health Encyclopedia*, New York: Van Nostrand Reinhold, 1981.
U.S. Department of Agriculture, *Handbook of the Nutritional Contents of Foods*, New York: Dover Publications, Inc., 1975.
Wurtman, Judith J., *Eating Your Way Through Life*, New York: Harper & Row, 1973.

Sources for vitamin section: *Earl Mindell's Vitamin Bible*, Earl Mindell, Rawson, Wade, Inc., New York, 1979, *Minerals and Your Health*, Len Mervyn, Ph.D., Keats Publishing Co., New Canaan, CT, 1980.

Measure	Calories Kcal	Protein g	Fat g	Carbohydrates g	Calcium mg	Iron mg	Sodium mg	Potassium mg	Vit. A mg	Thiamin IU	Riboflavin mg	Niacin mg	Vit. C mg
GRAINS													
Barley, pearled ½ cup cooked	98	2.3	.28	22	3	.59	1	36	-	.02	.01	.85	-
Buckwheat flour 1 cup sifted	340	6.4	1.1	78	11	1.0	1	314	-	.09	.05	.47	-
Cornmeal 1 cup dry	433	11	4.8	90	24	2.9	-	346	372	.46	.13	2.4	-
Millet ½ cup cooked	54	1.4	.5	11	3	1.1	1	64	-	.1	.06	.4	-
Oats, rolled ½ cup cooked	72.5	3	1.2	12.6	10	.8	.5	66	-	.13	.03	.15	-
Popcorn, plain 1 cup popped	23	.8	.3	4.6	1	.27	-	-	8	trace	.01	.1	-
Rice, brown ½ cup cooked	116	2.45	.78	25	13	.7	4.5	69	-	.09	.02	1.35	-
Soy flour, full-fat 1 cup sifted	295	26	14	31	143	5.4	1	1162	8	.6	.22	7.4	-
Wheat Bran 1 Tbsp.	5	36	.1	1.4	62	7.7	5	580	-	.37	.01	11	-
Wheat, bulghur ½ cup cooked	123	4.75	.48	22.1	14	1.4	1.5	76	-	.04	.03	2.05	-
Wheat flour 1 cup sifted	400	16	2	85	49	5.2	4	444	-	.66	.22	5.2	-
Wheat flour, pastry 1 cup sifted	496	14	-	110	53	4.4	4	580	0	.78	.18	7.8	-
Wheat germ 1 Tbsp.	17	1.25	.5	2.2	3.4	.28	.13	39	-	.09	.03	.2	-
LEGUMES													
Great Northern Beans 1 cup cooked	210	14	1.1	38	.9	4.1	5	726	-	.25	.13	.4	-
Kidney Beans 1 cup cooked	226	15	.9	41	53	6.6	4	710	10	.2	.11	1.2	-
Lentils 1 cup cooked	196	14	1	36	49	6.8	4	50	38	.14	.1	1.2	-
Lima Beans 1 cup cooked	270	16	1.2	50	52	5.9	4	1164	-	.26	.12	1.4	-
Mung Beans 1 cup cooked	141	10.6	.6	-	33	2.28	-	332	-	-	-	-	-
Navy Beans (Pea) 1 cup cooked	248	16	1.1	45	96	5	3	622	80	.27	.22	1.3	-
Peas, dried, split 1 cup cooked	230	16	.6	42	22	3.4	26	590	10	.3	.18	1.8	-
Pinto Beans 1 cup cooked	250	14.6	1	47	94	5.9	4	922	50	.5	.14	1.9	-
Soy Beans 1 cup cooked	234	20	10	20	132	6.9	4	970	50	.38	.15	1.1	-
Soy Grits 1 cup cooked	252	21	11	21	142	5.3	4.3	1050	54	.4	.16	1.2	-
Tempeh 2 oz.	117	11	5.1	3.4	48	1.9	.57	503	23	.08	.17	1.1	-
Tofu 2½"x2¾"x1"	86	9.4	5	3	154	2.2	8	50	-	.18	.08	.1	-
NUTS													
Almonds 12	106	3.25	9.6	3.5	42	.8	.6	137	-	.04	.16	.6	-
Brazil nuts 3 large	53	1.1	5.4	.9	15	.23	-	58	.86	.08	trace	.14	trace
Cashews 11 medium	98	3	8	5	6.6	1.1	2.6	81	17.5	.08	.04	.3	trace
Coconut, dried 1 cup shredded	493	5	49.5	11.5	19	3.9	19	522	-	.05	.03	.46	-
Filberts 11 nuts	95	1.9	9.7	2.5	34	1.2	.26	99	15	.07	.08	.13	-

	Measure	Calories Kcal	Protein g	Fat g	Carbohydrates g	Calcium mg	Iron mg	Sodium mg	Potassium mg	Vit. A mg	Thiamin IU	Riboflavin mg	Niacin mg	Vit. C mg
Peanuts, unsalted	2 Tbsp. chopped	106	4.7	9.2	2.5	12	.4	1.5	130	.3	.2	.02	3.2	-
Peanut butter	1 Tbsp.	94	4	7.8	3.6	11	.38	97	107	-	.06	.2	2.1	-
Pecans	2 Tbsp. chopped	101	1.4	10.5	2.1	11	.38	1.25	89	18.7	.13	.02	.14	.28
Pine Nuts	1 oz.	170	8.8	13.4	3.3	38	1.5	-	208	4	.25	.17	.95	-
Pistachios	2 Tbsp	105	3.4	9.4	3.4	23	1.2	.63	173	40	.12	.07	.25	-
Sesame Seeds, Whole	2 Tbsp	106	3.5	9.2	4	218	2	11	136	5.6	.18	.05	1	-
Sesame Seeds, Hulled	2 Tbsp	109	3.4	10	3.3	20.6	.46	8.8	142	1.5	.03	.02	1	-
Sunflower Seeds	2 Tbsp	101	4.4	8.6	3.6	22	1	5.4	167	8.8	.36	.04	1	-
Walnuts	2 Tbsp	98	2.2	9.6	2.4	15	.53	.25	68	5	.05	.02	.14	.29
VEGETABLES														
Avocados	3 ¼ diameter	457	5.6	43	21	31	2.8	30	1698	1735	.31	.3	5.4	22
Asparagus	1 cup cooked	29	3.2		5	30	1.5	8	309	1310	.23	.26	2	38
Beans, Green, Snap	1 cup cooked	31	.2	.25	7	63	1.2	5	370	680	.09	.11	.6	15
Beets	1 cup cooked	56	2.5	.2	12	34	1.3	73	530	30	.04	.07	.6	10
Beet Greens	1 cup cooked	23	1.8	.3	4	113	1.4	83	980	6092	.06	.17	.3	20
Broccoli	1 cup cooked	34	4.8	.5	5	132	1.2	16	324	3880	.13	.31	1.2	140
Brussel Sprouts	1 cup cooked	42	5.4	.6	6	50	1.5	15	372	715	.11	.19	1.2	135
Cabbage, shredded	1 cup cooked	26	2	.3	5	62	.4	16	234	247	.05	.05	.4	48
Carrots, diced	1 cup cooked	39	1.2	.3	9	48	.64	64	239	16280	.08	.07	.8	9
Cauliflower	1 cup cooked	20	2.5	.3	3	26	.6	13	400	59	.09	.09	.8	69
Chard, Swiss	1 cup cooked	31	3.2	.4	6	128	3.2	151	961	9450	.07	.2	.7	28
Collards	1 cup cooked	63	6.8	1.3	10	357	1.5	24	498	14820	.21	.38	2.3	144
Corn	½ cup cooked	89	3	1	21	2	.5	14	204	180	.18	.06	1.3	5
Cucumber	6 large slices	3	.2	trace	.7	5	.08	1.5	31	58	.01	.01	.08	2
Eggplant	1 cup cooked	38	2	.4	8.2	22	1.2	2	496	20	.1	.08	1	6
Kale	1 cup cooked	43	5	.8	7	206	1.8	47	244	9130	.11	.2	1.8	102
Lettuce, romaine	1 cup chopped	20	.7	.2	1.1	37	.6	4	99	.05	.03	.04	.2	10
Mushrooms	1 cup chopped	15	1.6	.3	3	4	1.2	7	256	-	.07	.3	2.9	2.5
Okra, sliced	1 cup cooked	46	3	.5	10	147	1.2	3	513	780	.21	.29	1.4	32
Onions, raw	1 cup chopped	60	3	.2	12	50	.8	15	231	35	.06	.07	.4	15
Parsnips	1 cup cooked	95	2.2	.8	22	70	.8	19	588	50	.11	.12	.2	16
Peas, green	1 cup cooked	99	8.3	.6	16	29	2.4	2	314	860	.43	.18	3.7	28

	Measure	Calories Kcal	Protein g	Fat g	Carbohydrates g	Calcium mg	Iron mg	Sodium mg	Potassium mg	Vit. A mg	Thiamin IU	Riboflavin mg	Niacin mg	Vit. C mg
Potatoes, boiled	1 med., in skin	105	2.9	.1	23	10	.8	4	556	trace	.12	.05	2	22
Spinach	¾ cup cooked	30	3.8	.38	4.5	125	3	71	437	10935	.1	.2	.67	38
Squash, summer	1 cup cooked	29	1.9	.2	7	53	.8	5	296	820	.1	.17	1.7	21
Squash, butternut	1 cup boiled	93	2.7	.7	23	49	1	2	632	8580	.1	.25	1.2	20
Tomatoes	1 medium	25	1	.2	6	16	.6	15	300	1110	.07	.05	.9	28
Tomato juice	1 cup canned	45	2	.2	10	17	2.2	696	552	1940	.12	.07	1.9	39
Turnips	1 cup cooked	35	1	.4	8	54	.6	48	29	trace	.06	.08	.5	34
FRUITS														
Apples	1 med, 3" diam.	81	.3	.5	21	10	.3	2	180	150	.05	.03	.2	7
Apple juice, unsweet.	1 cup	116	.2	.28	29	16	.9	5	296	trace	.05	.04	.25	2
Apple sauce, unsweet.	1 cup canned	106	.4	.12	28	7	.3	5	183	70	.03	.06	.46	3
Apricots, fresh	3	5	1.5	.4	12	15	.6	1	313	2769	.03	.04	.6	11
Bananas	1 medium	105	1.2	.5	27	7	.4	1	451	92	.05	.1	.6	10
Blueberries	1 cup raw	82	1	.5	21	9	.2	9	129	145	.07	.07	.7	19
Cantaloupe, half	5" diam.	80	2.5	.7	.8	28	.6	23	818	6921	.1	.07	1.5	89
Cherries, sweet	20	98	1.6	1.3	23	20	.5	.9	305	291	.07	.08	.5	10
Dates, dried, pitted	¼ cup chopped	122	.9	.2	33	15	.5	1.3	290	22	.04	.04	1	-
Figs, dried	2 medium	95	1.1	.4	24	54	.8	4	266	50	.03	.03	.3	trace
Grapefruit, half	4 " diam.	39	.8	.1	10	14	.07	-	175	12	.04	.02	.3	39
Grpefrt juice, fresh	1 cup unsweet	96	1.2	.2	23	22	.5	2	400	220	.1	.05	.5	94
Grapes, seedless	1 cup	114	1	.9	28	17	.4	3	296	117	.15	.09	.5	17
Grape juice, unsweet.	1 cup canned	155	1.4	.19	38	22	.6	8	334	20	.07	.09	.7	trace
Lemons	1 medium	17	.6	.2	5	15	.4	1	80	17	.02	.01	.06	31
Nectarines	1 medium	67	1.3	.6	16	6	.2	-	288	1001	.02	.06	1.4	7
Oranges	1 medium	62	1.2	.2	15	52	.14	-	237	269	.11	.05	.4	70
Ornge juice, unsweet	1 cup fresh	111	1.7	.5	26	27	.3	2	496	496	.22	.07	1	124
Peach, peeled	1 medium	37	.6	.08	10	5	.1	1	171	465	.02	.04	.8	6
Pear	1 medium	98	.7	.7	25	19	.4	1	208	33	.03	.07	.2	7
Pineapple	1 cup, diced	77	.6	.7	20	11	.6	1	175	35	.14	.06	.7	24
Plums, fresh	3 whole 2" diam.	119	1.7	1.4	28	6.6	.23	-	373	704	.01	.02	1	21
Prunes, dried	5 large, uncooked	117	1.5	.3	31	25	1.2	1.8	365	974	.04	.08	1	trace
Raisins	¼ cup	124	1.3	.2	33	20	.9	4.8	310	trace	.06	.04	.34	trace

	Measure	Calories Kcal	Protein g	Fat g	Carbohydrates g	Calcium mg	Iron mg	Sodium mg	Potassium mg	Vit. A mg	Thiamin IU	Riboflavin mg	Niacin mg	Vit. C mg
Strawberries	1 cup whole	45	1	.6	11	21	.6	2	247	41	.03	.1	.34	85
Watermelon	1 cup diced	50	1	.7	12	13	.3	3	186	585	.13	.03	.3	15
DAIRY														
Cheddar, American	2 inch cube	133	7.9	10.6	.56	233	.13	508	43	429	.01	.13	.02	-
Cottage, low-fat	1 cup	204	31	4.4	8	135	.36	914	218	158	.05	.4	.3	-
Cream Cheese	2 Tbsp	99	2	9.5	.75	44	.39	84	33	405	trace	.06	.03	-
Edam	2 inch cube	126	9	9.8	.5	259	.17	343	51	325	.01	.14	.03	-
Parmesan, grated	1 Tbsp	23	2.1	1.5	trace	70	.05	9.4	6	36	trace	.02	.02	-
Swiss, American	2 inch cube	134	10	9.4	1.2	340	.2	93	38	300	trace	.13	.03	-
Cream, light	2 Tbsp	59	.8	6	1	29	.01	12	37	216	trace	.04	.02	trace
Eggs, raw	1 large	79	6	5.6	trace	28	1	59	65	260	.04	.15	-	-
Milk, buttermilk	1 cup	99	8	2.1	12	285	1	257	371	81	.08	.38	.14	2
Milk, nonfat instant	1 cup, dry	244	24	.5	36	857	.2	373	1160	1612	.28	1.2	.6	3.8
Milk, 2% low-fat	1 cup	121	8	4.9	12	297	1	122	377	500	.1	.4	.2	2
Milk, skim	1 cup	86	8.4	.4	12	302	.1	126	406	500	.09	.34	.2	2
Milk, whole	1 cup	150	8	8	11	291	.1	12	370	307	.09	.4	.2	2
Yogurt, skim	1 cup	127	13	.4	17	452	.2	174	579	50	.10	.53	.3	2
Yogurt, whole	1 cup, plain	139	7.9	7.4	11	274	.1	105	351	680	.07	.32	.2	1
FATS														
Butter, salted	1 Tbsp	102	.1	11.5	trace	3.37	.02	117	3.6	434	-	trace	trace	0
Margarine	1 Tbsp	102	.13	11.4	.13	375	.02	134	3	469	-	-	-	0
Oil, corn	1 Tbsp	120	0	14	0	0	0	0	0	.06	0	0	0	0
Oil, peanut or olive	1 Tbsp	119	0	14	0	0	0	0	0	-	0	0	0	0
Mayonaise	1 Tbsp	99	.2	11	trace	2.5	.07	78	5	39	trace	.01	trace	0
MISCELLANEOUS														
Honey	1 Tbsp	64.4	.062	0	17.4	1	1.1	-	23	0	trace	.01	.06	.19
Molasses, light	1 Tbsp	43	-	-	11	33	1.1	3	183	-	.01	.01	.01	-
Molasses, blackstrap	1 Tbsp	50	-	-	15	157	4.4	19	585	-	.02	.04	.4	-
Yeast, Nutritional, Brewers	1 Tbsp	23	3.1	.1	3	17	1.4	10	144	1	1.3	.34	3.2	trace

*Values for these tables were reprinted by permission from *The New Laurel's Kitchen*, by Laurel Robertson, Carol Flinders and Brian Ruppenthal, copyright 1986, Ten Speed Press, Berkeley, California

Index